Evolution of Department Defense Disability Evaluation and Management of Posttraumatic Stress Disorder and Traumatic Brain Injury

T0119353

Overview of Policy Changes, 2001–2018

MOLLY M. SIMMONS, CARRIE M. FARMER, SAMANTHA CHERNEY, HEATHER KRULL

Prepared for the U.S. Department of Defense Psychological Health Center of Excellence
Approved for public release; distribution unlimited

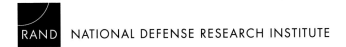 NATIONAL DEFENSE RESEARCH INSTITUTE

For more information on this publication, visit www.rand.org/t/RR3173

Library of Congress Cataloging-in-Publication Data is available for this publication.
ISBN: 978-1-9774-0502-9

Published by the RAND Corporation, Santa Monica, Calif.
© Copyright 2021 RAND Corporation
RAND® is a registered trademark.

Cover image: U.S. Army photo

Support RAND
Make a tax-deductible charitable contribution at
www.rand.org/giving/contribute

www.rand.org

Preface

Service members whose illnesses or injuries call into question their ability to fulfill their military duties may be referred by a health care provider to the Integrated Disability Evaluation System (IDES), a joint program of the U.S. Department of Defense (DoD) and the U.S. Department of Veterans Affairs (VA). This program is responsible for determining whether the individual is fit for duty as guided by his or her military department standards and requirements. If the service member is found to be unfit, he or she is medically discharged from military service. The process also assesses the extent to which the individual is considered to be disabled and assigns a rating, which in turns helps to determine what type of disability compensation he or she may be due. Since 2001, there have been several changes to DoD and VA disability evaluation policies and processes. Most notably, in 2007, the departments moved away from conducting their own respective medical evaluations and ratings and toward an integrated system. During this same period, there were also numerous policy changes related to screening, diagnosing, and treating what have become known as the "signature injuries" of the wars in Iraq and Afghanistan: posttraumatic stress disorder (PTSD) and traumatic brain injury (TBI).

The DoD Psychological Health Center of Excellence asked the RAND Corporation to assess trends in DoD disability evaluation policies and disability benefits for PTSD and TBI. The study documented changes in policy and practice since 2001, historical trends in disability evaluations and outcomes, contemporaneous trends in the diagnosis and treatment of PTSD and TBI, the context in which service members are evaluated for disabilities associated with these conditions, and the process for conducting these evaluations. This report describes RAND's review of disability evaluation system (DES) policies and changes in the diagnosis and treatment of PTSD and TBI since 2001. A companion report (Krull et al., 2021) presents RAND's analyses of trends in disability evaluations and treatment for service members with PTSD and/or TBI since 2001. The research reported here was completed in August 2019 and underwent security review with the sponsor and the Defense Office of Prepublication and Security Review before public release.

This research was sponsored by the Psychological Health Center of Excellence and conducted within the Forces and Resources Policy Center of the RAND National Security Research Division (NSRD), which operates the National Defense Research Institute (NDRI), a federally funded research and development center sponsored by the Office of the Secretary of Defense, the Joint Staff, the Unified Combatant Commands, the Navy, the Marine Corps, the defense agencies, and the defense intelligence enterprise.

For more information on the RAND Forces and Resources Policy Center, see www.rand.org/nsrd/frp or contact the director (contact information is provided on the webpage).

Contents

Figures and Table

Figures

Table

Summary

Since 2001, the United States has been engaged in continuous combat operations in Iraq, Afghanistan, and other theaters. Many service members have sustained injuries or developed medical conditions as a consequence of combat or military service and are thus no longer able to serve. The process by which the U.S. Department of Defense (DoD) evaluates service members and determines whether they should be medically discharged has changed considerably since 2001; major changes to the disability evaluation system (DES), in particular, were implemented beginning in 2007. Simultaneously, DoD also implemented new policies in response to what have become known as "signature injuries" of the wars in Iraq and Afghanistan: posttraumatic stress disorder (PTSD) and traumatic brain injury (TBI). This report reviews major policy changes to DES between 2001 and 2018 with a particular focus on changes to policies related to the screening and treatment of PTSD and TBI. A companion report (Krull et al., 2021) presents an analysis of how rates of diagnoses for these conditions and referrals to DES have changed over the same time period (i.e., 2001 to 2018).

Service members who become wounded, ill, or injured while serving may seek and receive treatment for up to one year following diagnosis, or until further recovery is relatively predictable, whichever comes first. If at that point service members' medical condition(s) prevents them from performing the duties of their office, grade, rank, or rating, or if the medical condition(s) poses a risk to them, a medical provider may refer them for disability and retention evaluation (Department of Defense Instruction [DoDI] 1332.18, 2016). After being referred, the service member begins with a medical exam that is conducted by the U.S. Department of Veterans Affairs (VA). Then, the DoD medical evaluation board (MEB) determines if the service member meets medical retention standards according to his or her branch of service. If MEB finds that the service member meets medical retention standards, he or she is returned to duty. If the service member does not meet medical retention standards, the case is forwarded to the DoD physical evaluation board (PEB) to determine if the service member is fit for duty—meaning that despite any medical conditions, the service member is still able to do his or her job. Service members who are found fit for duty are returned to duty; service members who are found unfit have their cases forwarded to VA, where every medical condition identified in the medical exam is assigned a disability rating. Compensation from DoD includes only those conditions that make the service member unfit for duty in its rating, whereas VA compensates for all service-related conditions identified in the medical exam. Unfit service members are then medically separated or retired, and disability benefits, for those eligible to receive them, begin within 30 days of discharge.

Disability Evaluation Policy Changes Since 2007

Prior to 2007, service members were evaluated and, if necessary, medically discharged through DoD's DES. Discharged service members then applied for disability and health care benefits from VA and were evaluated a second time by VA. Because DoD and VA conducted separate evaluations, according to different criteria, the disability determination would often differ, which created inefficiencies and confusion for transitioning service members.

In 2007, a *Washington Post* article raised questions about the housing conditions and quality of care for service members being treated for combat-related conditions at Walter Reed Army Medical Center (Priest and Hull, 2007). The investigation came on the heels of high-profile media accounts of the psychological toll of deployments to Iraq and

Afghanistan. In response to this confluence of events, DoD, Congress, and the George W. Bush administration launched investigations, task forces, and commissions to determine the evaluation and treatment needs of service members returning from the global War on Terror—including the efficiency and consistency of DES. To provide oversight and coordination of the various commissions and groups examining wounded warrior issues, the Secretaries of Veterans Affairs and Defense established the Wounded, Ill, and Injured Senior Oversight Committee (SOC) in 2007 (VA and DoD, 2009). Collectively, these groups called for significant changes to the disability evaluation process. For example,

- The President's Commission on Care for America's Returning Wounded Warriors was established by President George W. Bush to examine the care provided to returning service members "from the time they leave the battlefield through their return to civilian life" (President's Commission, 2007). Among other recommendations, the final report recommended significantly restructuring and simplifying the DoD and VA disability and compensation systems.
- An Independent Review Group commissioned by the Secretary of Defense to review rehabilitative care and administrative processes at Walter Reed Army Medical Center and the National Naval Medical Center recommended the establishment of a center of excellence for the treatment of PTSD and TBI and a complete overhaul of DES (Independent Review Group, 2007).
- The Veterans Disability Benefits Commission was established to examine and assess how VA compensated veterans for service-connected disabilities and deaths. Its final report showed that the evaluation system was confusing, even to some raters, and that changes were needed (Christensen et al., 2007). A related Institute of Medicine (IOM) Committee report recommended changes to the Veterans Affairs Schedule for Rating Disabilities (VASRD), including a recommendation that it compensate for not only lost earnings but also nonwork disability and loss of quality of life (McGeary et al., 2007).

The National Defense Authorization Act (NDAA) for fiscal year (FY) 2008 authorized DoD to launch pilot programs to improve the DES, laying the groundwork for the Integrated Disability Evaluation System (IDES) (Pub. L. 110-181, §1644). Incorporating the recommendations of the various commissions and task forces, DoD and VA jointly launched a pilot program to evaluate whether VA should conduct medical exams during the disability evaluation process, with DoD maintaining control over the determination of ability to serve. The goal of the pilot was to reduce processing times and redundancies in the system, as well as eliminate variation across military branches. The program successfully demonstrated the efficiency of integrated processes and was officially adopted in 2011.

As required by other language in the FY2008 NDAA, DoD directed the strict adoption of the VASRD DoD-wide. Disability ratings are consequential for service members because they serve as the basis for qualification for medical retirement. With the adoption of VASRD, service members who are determined to be unfit because of "mental health disorders due to traumatic stress" (e.g., PTSD) receive a minimum 50 percent disability rating and are placed on the Temporary Disability Retired List (TDRL) and reevaluated within six months. Previously, service members who were found unfit because of PTSD were assigned a disability rating based on functional impairment.

Policy Changes Specific to Posttraumatic Stress Disorder and Traumatic Brain Injury

Since the start of the conflicts in Iraq and Afghanistan, significant changes in our understanding of PTSD and TBI have resulted in policy changes within the military health system. As studies highlighted an increase in the prevalence of PTSD and TBI among service members who had deployed to combat zones (Hoge et al., 2004; Milliken et al., 2007; Tanielian et al., 2008), the presidential and DoD commissions that led to changes in DES also recommended that additional attention and resources be devoted to detecting and treating PTSD, TBI, and mental health issues in general.

In response, DoD implemented numerous programs, initiatives, and new policies designed to increase detection of these conditions and ensure that service members received high-quality treatment. Service members who deploy to a theater of combat are now required to complete health assessments both before and after a deployment. These required assessments are a valuable tool for tracking PTSD, TBI, and other mental health conditions.

After the implementation of IDES and the revised VASRD policy, there were still concerns about whether service members with PTSD were receiving accurate disability evaluations. In 2008, a group of veterans filed a class action lawsuit alleging that the PEB had not adhered to the 50 percent disability rating standard (*Sabo v. United States*, 2011). That same year, Army Medical Command found that providers at one military treatment facility (MTF) had changed service members' diagnoses to something other than PTSD due to suspicion that service members were exaggerating their PTSD symptoms to qualify for disability benefits (Moisse, 2012; Ashton, 2013a). An investigation of another military installation revealed that service members who exhibited behavioral health problems associated with TBI and PTSD after being exposed to traumatic events were being given less-than-honorable discharges (Zwerdling, 2015). In response to these events, there was a broad re-review of disability cases for service members whose disability ratings or determinations had been called into question.

Conclusion

While DES has been in existence since 1947, the period from 2001 to 2018 was characterized by particularly significant changes—not only in DES itself but also in the understanding and treatment of PTSD and TBI. A companion report (Krull et al., 2021) describes trends in diagnoses of PTSD and TBI over this same period, along with trends in disability evaluation outcomes, such as disability ratings and final dispositions. This report provides context for considering those trends, potential additional initiatives and policy changes, and the implications of the new landscape for assessing and evaluating these signature injuries of the Iraq and Afghanistan wars.

Acknowledgments

We gratefully acknowledge the support of our current and previous project sponsors, CAPT Carrie Kennedy, Dr. Marjorie Campbell, and CAPT Michael Colston, as well as the staff at the Psychological Health Centers of Excellence, especially Maria Morgan. We also thank several individuals who have knowledge of the history and policy evolution of DES, including Al Bruner with Health Services Policy and Oversight; Jimmy (JD) Stevens, Tammy Hern, and the rest of the Air Force DES Quality Assurance team; Frances Dennis at the Army Physical Disability Agency; John Fitzpatrick and other staff at the Navy Physical Evaluation Board; and Susan Hosek at RAND. The input provided by these individuals was invaluable and informed the analyses and interpretations described in this report. They are not responsible for the contents of this report or the recommendations contained herein. We thank Lauren Skrabala for her writing and editing support and Stephanie Lonsinger, Brittany Joseph, and Lee Remi for their assistance in preparing this report. Finally, we are grateful to Terri Tanielian at RAND and Tim Hoyt at the Defense Health Agency for serving as technical peer reviewers; their comments greatly improved this report.

Abbreviations

ASD(HA)	Assistant Secretary of Defense for Health Affairs
ATFBH	Army Task Force on Behavioral Health
C&P	compensation and pension
CAP	corrective action plan
CFR	Code of Federal Regulations
CRSC	combat-related special compensation
DCoE	Defense Centers of Excellence
DD	Department of Defense
DES	disability evaluation system
DoD	Department of Defense
DoDI	Department of Defense Instruction
D-RAS	Disability Evaluation System Rating Activity Site
DSM	*Diagnostic and Statistical Manual*
DTM	directive-type memorandum
EDES	Expedited Disability Evaluation System
FPEB	Formal Physical Evaluation Board
FY	fiscal year
GAO	Government Accountability Office
IDES	Integrated Disability Evaluation System
IOM	Institute of Medicine
IPDES	Integrated Pilot Disability Evaluation System

IPEB	Informal Physical Evaluation Board
LDES	Legacy Disability Evaluation System
LOA	line of action
MACE	Military Acute Concussion Evaluation
MEB	medical evaluation board
MHA	mental health assessment
MHAT	Mental Health Advisory Team
MOA	memorandum of agreement
MTF	military treatment facility
NDAA	National Defense Authorization Act
OEF	Operation Enduring Freedom
OIF	Operation Iraqi Freedom
P&R	personnel and readiness
PC-PTSD	Primary Care PTSD Screen
PDBR	Physical Disability Board of Review
PDHA	Post-Deployment Health Assessment
PDHRA	Post-Deployment Health Reassessment
PEB	physical evaluation board
PEBLO	Physical Evaluation Board Liaison Officer
Pre-DHA	Pre-Deployment Health Assessment
PTSD	posttraumatic stress disorder
SOC	Senior Oversight Committee
TBI	traumatic brain injury
TDRL	Temporary Disability Retired List
VA	U.S. Department of Veterans Affairs
UCMJ	Uniform Code of Military Justice
VASRD	Veterans Affairs Schedule for Rating Disabilities

CHAPTER ONE

Introduction and Overview

Since 2001, the United States has been engaged in continuous combat operations in Afghanistan, Iraq, and other theaters, and over three million service members have deployed in support of these operations (Defense Manpower Data Center, 2018). As a consequence of combat and military service, many service members have experienced physical and mental injuries (DoD, 2019; Mann, 2019), including posttraumatic stress disorder (PTSD) and traumatic brain injury (TBI), which have come to be known as the signature injuries from the global War on Terror (Tanielian and Jaycox, 2008). PTSD is a mental health condition that some people experience after a terrifying or life-threatening event, such as combat. People with PTSD often experience nightmares, flashbacks, and intense anxiety, with symptoms lasting for months (VA, 2019a), or for some patients, throughout their lives. There are effective treatments for PTSD, so ensuring that service members with PTSD are identified and treated is a priority for the military health system. TBI is a serious head injury that causes temporary or permanent damage to the brain. A TBI can be mild, moderate, or severe. Mild TBIs, also known as concussions, are the most common type of TBIs (CDC, 2019). Recovery from TBI depends greatly on the severity of the injury; most of those with a mild TBI have a complete recovery.

While many service members with PTSD or TBI receive treatment, recover, and return to duty, those who are unable to make a full recovery are referred to the disability evaluation system (DES) to be evaluated for medical discharge. In recent years, over 20,000 service members have been medically discharged and separated from military service each year through DES (Boivin et al., 2015).

DES has changed considerably between 2001 and 2018, due in part to larger disability evaluation caseloads during this time as the number of service members with deployment-related injuries and illnesses has increased. Over the same time period, PTSD and TBI have been recognized as signature injuries from the contemporaneous wars, and numerous policies related to the identification and treatment of these conditions have been implemented (Blakeley and Jansen, 2013). The Department of Defense (DoD) Centers of Excellence for Psychological Health and Traumatic Brain Injury,[1] which was established in 2007 as part of DoD's efforts to improve care for these signature injuries, asked RAND to review and describe major policy changes related to DES and the identification and treatment of PTSD and TBI as part of a study of trends in service members' diagnoses, treatment, and disability referrals and evaluations for PTSD or TBI. This report reviews how DES has changed between 2001and 2018 and describes policy changes related to screening and treatment of PTSD and TBI. A companion report (Krull et al., 2021) analyzes changes between 2001 and 2018 in the rates of diagnosis, treatment, and disability evaluations for service members with PTSD and/or TBI.

Methods

The goal of this analysis was to identify and review the major policy changes between 2001 and 2018 related to the DES, as well as to review major policy changes associated with the identification and treatment of PTSD and TBI among service members. We began by searching DoD and the U.S. Department of Veterans Affairs (VA) publication websites to identify official policy documents and reports, using search terms such as "PTSD," "TBI" (individually and in combination), "disability evaluation," "mental health," "medical evaluation board," and "physical evaluation board." We also identified and reviewed any refer-

---

[1]   In 2017, the Defense Centers of Excellence for Psychological Health and Traumatic Brain Injury was reorganized into separate centers within the Defense Health Agency. The sponsoring office for this study became the Psychological Health Center of Excellence.

ences referred to in these documents to identify sources we may have missed, as well as older documents, including those that might have since been superseded. Some of these were publicly available, while others required access to restricted sites, including the Defense Technical Information Center.[2] We also reviewed various websites, such as the DoD Office of Warrior Care Policy, for additional sources. With a few exceptions, our analysis focused on DoD policies rather than on policies issued by individual service branches.

To locate statutes and federal regulations, we reviewed the references in the most relevant DoD documents. After finding those statutes and regulations on LexisNexis, we examined prior versions of the law. We also made sure to review the other sections in the chapters where we found relevant laws. We reviewed the National Defense Authorization Acts (NDAA) from 2001 to 2017, selecting the sections referencing TBI, PTSD, and disability evaluation. We expanded our investigation of these NDAAs to include relevant reports and briefings. We also reviewed important case law. In addition, we reviewed government reports, newspaper articles, and other documents that provided context for policy changes.

Finally, we hosted meetings with stakeholders in DoD and the service branches. We spoke to policymakers, as well as those who oversee the execution of DES. During those meetings, we discussed our review of policy changes and asked individuals to help us identify any we may have missed or to share copies of documents that we were unable to locate through our traditional search methods. Stakeholders were also able to provide some background on the impetus for many policy changes.

---

[2] Access to the restricted Defense Technical Information Center portal requires a Common Access Card.

CHAPTER TWO

Evolution of the Disability Evaluation System

The federal government has been involved in the care and compensation of American service members permanently disabled in service to their country since the inception of the United States (VDBC, 2007; Rostker, 2013). In 1776, the Continental Congress voted to compensate any soldier injured in battle in defense of the colony, and over the next 250 years, the federal government's management of disabled service members separating from the military evolved considerably. In this chapter, we describe the current "mechanism for the retirement or separation of a military member due to physical disability" (Marcum et al., 2002), known as the Integrated Disability Evaluation System (IDES). We explain how the system works today, provide a history of how this process was created, and detail the changes that have been made over time. A timeline of these changes and history is presented in Table 2.1.

The Disability Evaluation Process

IDES is the current process used to evaluate a service member's medical conditions and determine eligibility for medical retirement or separation with or without severance pay (DoD Warrior Care, undated). Prior to IDES, DoD followed a process now referred to as the Legacy

5

Disability Evaluation System (LDES).[1] The key elements of both the LDES and the current IDES process include

- medical examination
- medical evaluation board (MEB) evaluations
- physical evaluation board (PEB) evaluations and appellate review
- member counseling
- final disposition.

When a service member is referred for disability evaluation, he or she receives a medical examination, during which a physician identifies all service-connected health conditions. After the exam, the service member's case is reviewed by MEB. Each military installation with a medical facility has an MEB, which is composed of several physicians. MEB uses information from the medical exam, medical records, and a service member's commander to determine whether the service member has a medical condition that results in the service member being unable to meet medical retention standards set by military regulations. MEB then forwards its decisions to PEB. Each service branch has a PEB, which is composed of a mix of officers and physicians. PEB determines whether the service member's medical conditions are unfitting, meaning the service member is no longer able to fulfill the duties of his or her military occupation and rank. For medical conditions that are unfitting, PEB also determines whether the condition(s) is stable and whether or not it is compensable (Department of Defense Instruction [DoDI] 1332.18, 2014, p. 31). *Compensable* means the service member's injuries or illnesses are eligible for disability compensation. If MEB determines that the service member meets medical retention standards, or if PEB determines that the service member's conditions do not make him or her unfit for service, the service member is returned to duty.

---

[1]   Throughout this report, we will use the following terminology: DES refers generally to disability evaluation, including both the current IDES and LDES; LDES refers to the primary system used prior to 2012, when IDES was fully implemented across DoD; IDES refers to the primary system used since 2012 when the DoD and VA disability evaluations were fully integrated. The LDES is still used in certain circumstances and if we refer to it after 2012, the year is noted. Between 2007 and 2011, pilots of an integrated system were conducted, so there is overlap between LDES as the primary system and IDES.

As part of the PEB process, service members with unfitting conditions receive a disability rating for each condition to reflect the severity of the disability. Under LDES, DoD conducted the medical examination and assigned disability ratings for each unfitting condition. Then, after separating from the military, the individual went through a separate evaluation process by VA and received a VA disability rating. It was often the case that DoD and VA disability ratings were different, which caused confusion and frustration. In IDES, VA conducts the medical examination. Every medical condition identified in the medical exam is assigned a disability rating by the VA. Compensation from DoD includes only those conditions that make the service member unfit for duty in its rating, whereas VA includes compensation for all service-related conditions identified in the medical exam.

The disability rating is based on the criteria found in the Veterans Affairs Schedule for Rating Disabilities (VASRD) publication (DoDI 1332.39, 1996, p. 3; 38 CFR, Subpart B, Disability Ratings, Sections 4.40-4.130, 1996). Disability ratings range from 0 to 100 percent, in 10 percent increments, where 0 percent means the condition is not serious and the service member can work and perform activities of daily living without any problems, and 100 percent means the service member is completely disabled, unable to work or perform in a social setting. The disability ratings for each unfitting condition are combined into a total disability rating, which is used to determine the final outcome of the disability evaluation process.

Following determination of the total combined disability rating, a service member receives a final disposition, which could be one of the following:

- *Medical Separation*: Service members with a total combined disability rating of 0, 10, or 20 percent and less than 20 years of service are separated from the military and receive six months of health care benefits and a lump-sum severance payment commensurate with their length of service.
- *Medical Retirement*: Service members with a total combined disability rating of 30 percent or higher (or 20 years of service) are medically retired, which means that they receive monthly disabil-

ity pay for life (paid by both DoD and VA[2]), as well as lifetime health care benefits.

- *Separated without Benefits*: Service members with disabling conditions that the PEB determines existed prior to military service and were not service aggravated are separated without benefits. This same outcome results if PEB determines that the condition(s) were the result of the service member's own misconduct.

Service members who are medically retired are either permanently retired due to disability or temporarily retired due to disability. Service members who have medical conditions that have not stabilized—for example, PTSD—are temporarily retired, which means that they initially receive monthly cash and health care benefits, and are periodically reevaluated. If reevaluation finds that the service member has recovered or the severity of the condition has lessened, the final disability rating and separation type (retirement or medical separation) may change. In rare cases, a service member may be found to have recovered sufficiently to be returned to duty.

For the establishment of permanent disability, and therefore retirement from the military as a result of that disability with no further reevaluation, the injury/illness must be considered "permanent and stable" and not be due to the service member's "neglect, misconduct" or incurred "during unauthorized absence" (10 U.S.C. §1201, 2008; DoDI 1332.38, 1996).

Service members have a number of opportunities to appeal their disposition. For example, following MEB, service members can request to have an impartial physician review their medical evidence and present a rebuttal to the MEB findings. After PEB, which first meets

---

[2] DoD's disability compensation paid to retirees is offset dollar-for-dollar by VA disability compensation, which is also based on the service member's disability rating. However, service members with combat-related disabilities, who are entitled to disability or nondisability retired pay from DoD and who have at least a 10 percent disability rating from VA may apply for Combat Related Special Compensation (CRSC). If approved, they are entitled to receive nontaxable monthly payments. CRSC was established as part of the 2003 NDAA (Pub. L. 107-314) and was expanded in the 2004 and 2008 NDAAs (Pub. L. 108-136 and Pub. L. 110-181, respectively).

informally to make a determination, a service member can request a formal PEB. Following the formal PEB decision, the service member can appeal to have the case be reviewed by his or her service appellate review authority.

Establishment of the Integrated Disability Evaluation System

As a consequence of the wars in Iraq and Afghanistan, the number of service members wounded or injured in combat rose significantly after 2001. The care and treatment of these returning service members was a focus of much media reporting during the early years of the wars, with multiple news reports investigating substandard care (Benjamin, 2003), high rates of mental health problems (Welch, 2005), and questions about how service members with war-related disabilities were faring (Hull, 2004).

There were also concerns raised about DES specifically. A 2002 RAND study (Marcum et al., 2002) found variability in DES policy application across the Army, Navy, and Air Force. In 2006, the Government Accountability Office (GAO) similarly reported inconsistencies in disability evaluation processes across the services and a lack of DoD-level standardization and oversight (GAO, 2006). Research showed many service members felt that receiving a disability rating from both DoD and VA was confusing and found the dual adjudication slow and difficult to navigate (President's Commission, 2007, p. 25). Some of the confusion may have been because VA benefits are based on disability from all medical conditions determined to have arisen or been aggravated during military service, whereas DoD benefits are based only on those conditions that are unfitting for military service. However, there were also inconsistencies between DoD and VA determinations, such as the VA rating exceeding the DoD rating for a given condition, which was often the case for PTSD and TBI (IOM, 2007a, p. 115). While other issues further added to the confusion, as early as 2003 there were official recommendations to move to a single discharge medical exam as opposed to the dual adjudication system to try to lessen confusion and increase consistency (President's Task Force, 2003, pp. 29–30).[3]

In 2006, to provide support for service members who were navigating the disability evaluation process, the 2007 National Defense Authorization Act (NDAA) mandated training requirements and standardized procedures for case officers, called PEB Liaison Officers (PEBLOs) (Pub. L. 109-364, Sub. C, §597, Physical Evaluation Boards, 2006). PEBLOs help service members navigate the PEB process and secure legal counsel for service members who wished to appeal their decision (DoD OUSD [Personnel and Readiness (P&R)], 2008, pp. 3–6).

Public attention to the treatment and evaluation of wounded service members grew with reports of problems and concerns for this population. In February 2007, the *Washington Post* published a series of articles detailing concerning conditions and patient treatment at Walter Reed Army Medical Center (Priest and Hull, 2007). The *Washington Post* story proved to be a tipping point, and the resulting public outcry led to numerous investigations, commissions, reports, and, ultimately, significant policy changes, including a transformation of DES (see Table 2.1). In the sections that follow, we describe this evolution.

2007: Formally Setting the Stage for Changes to the Disability Evaluation System

While changes to DES may have happened without the *Washington Post* story, that story focused what was already consistent pressure from veterans' organizations and news media on a single issue. Congressional staff cited the articles as a catalyst to make changes to the disability system (Simmons, 2015, p. 54). In March 2007, President George W. Bush visited Water Reed, and in remarks to the hospital staff he noted, "The problems at Walter Reed were caused by bureaucratic and administrative failures. The system failed you, and it failed our troops. And

---

[3] U.S. Government Accountability Office, *Progress Made on Implementation of 2003 President's Task Force Recommendations on Collaboration and Coordination, but More Remains to Be Done*, Washington, D.C.,[0][0] GAO 08-495R, April 30, 2008, states that a recommendation was made to "implement a mandatory single physical examination for servicemembers separating from military service and electronic transmission of separation information."

Table 2.1
Timeline of Significant Events Transforming the Disability Evaluation System

Year	Event
2002	• RAND Report found variability in DES application across services (Marcum et al., 2002, p. 1).
2003	• GAO 08-495R recommended that DoD "implement a mandatory single physical examination for servicemembers separating from military service and electronic transmission of separation information."
	• President's Task Force to Improve Health Care Delivery for Our Nation's Veterans, *Final Report*, was published in May 2003.
	• Veterans Disability Benefits Commission established by the 2004 NDAA.
2006	• GAO reported inconsistencies in disability evaluation processes across the services and a lack of DoD-level standardization and oversight.
	• The 2007 NDAA included a requirement for PEBLO, a new role of case officer.
2007	• In February 2007, the *Washington Post* published a series of articles detailing concerning conditions and patient treatment at Walter Reed Army Medical Center (Priest and Hull, 2007).
	• President Bush created the Commission on Care for America's Returning Wounded Warriors (commonly called the Dole-Shalala Commission after its two chairs).
	• Defense Secretary Robert M. Gates created an Independent Review Group, also known as the Marsh-West Group, to review the care and administrative processes at Walter Reed and the National Naval Medical Center.
	• In August the Veterans Disability Benefits Commission delivered its report, which found that the current rating system was confusing even to raters in some categories. It also noted that ratings were higher from the VA than they were for the DoD both on the number of conditions that were rated and the level at which individual conditions were rated.
	• An Institute of Medicine (IOM) report recommended changes to VASRD, including a recommendation that it compensate not only for lost earnings but also for nonwork disability and loss of quality of life.
	• The Secretaries of Veterans Affairs and Defense established the Wounded, Ill and Injured Senior Oversight Committee (SOC).
	• Congress passed the "Dignified Treatment of Wounded Warriors Act," which included provisions to evaluate and alter the disability system.
	• The 2008 NDAA established major changes to DES and laid the groundwork for the move to IDES, including an IDES pilot authorization.
	• The IDES pilot launched at three sites.

Table 2.1—Continued

Year	Event
2008	○ "Policy Memorandum on Implementing Disability-Related Provisions of the National Defense Authorization Act of 2008" (Pub 1. 110-181) was published and ○ Rescinded DoDI 1332.39, 1996 (Application of the Veterans Administration Schedule for Rating Disabilities) and directed military departments to use only the VASRD ratings. In addition, DoDI 1332.38, 1996, was updated with policy from the now-rescinded DoDI 1332.39. ○ Required that service members who were determined to be unfit because of "mental health disorders due to traumatic stress" (e.g., PTSD) were to receive a minimum 50 percent disability rating and be placed on the Temporary Disability Retired List (TDRL) and reevaluated within six months (unless their total disability rating was 80 percent or higher, in which case they should be permanently retired). ○ Established timeline goals for each step in the disability process. ○ Altered the procedures for service members' review of their disability determinations. • Department of Defense, Under Secretary of Defense (Personnel Readiness), "Directive-Type Memorandum (DTM) 11-015—Policy and Procedural Update for the Disability Evaluation System (DES) Pilot Program," was published on December 11, 2008. • Memorandum of agreement (MOA) was established between VA and DoD on IDES scope, policy, responsibilities and implementing instructions.
2009	• The 2010 NDAA required that the services assess the impact of a PTSD or TBI diagnosis on service members prior to administratively discharging them for misconduct. • MOA between the VA and DoD expanded the number of IDES pilot sites by 2010 to 24 sites. • Department of Defense, Under Secretary of Defense (Personnel and Readiness) published a memorandum to establish the Expedited Disability Evaluation System (EDES): Expedited DES Process for Members with Catastrophic Conditions and Combat-Related Stress.
2010	• A GAO report found average time a service member waited for adjudication was cut almost in half under the Integrated Pilot Disability Evaluation System (IPDES) compared with the DES.
2011	• Department of Defense, Under Secretary of Defense (Personnel and Readiness), "Directive-Type Memorandum 11-015 Integrated Disability Evaluation System (IDES)," was revised to formally establish IDES.
2014	• DoDI 1332.14 *Enlisted Administrative Separations* was published and disallowed separation for a personality disorder or other mental disorder not constituting a physical disability if service-related PTSD is also diagnosed. It also required an examination for PTSD or TBI if service member was being administratively separated, was deployed to a contingency operation during previous 24 months, or was diagnosed with PTSD, as well as if separation was not pursuant to a court martial or Uniform Code of Military Justice (UCMJ) proceeding.

Table 2.1—Continued

Year	Event
2015	• DoDI 6040.44, *Physical Disability Board of Review*, was published and established policies, assigned responsibilities, and provided procedures for Physical Disability Board of Review (PDBR) operation and management as required by Section 1554a of U.S. Code, Title 10. It also designated the Secretary of the Air Force as the lead agent for the establishment, operation, and management of the PDBR for DoD.
	• Department of Defense, Under Secretary of Defense (Personnel and Readiness), "Memorandum: Enrollment in the Legacy Disability Evaluation System," was published and perpetuated LDES for service members by request.
2016	• The 2017 NDAA amended U.S. Code, Title 10, Section 1210, reducing the maximum time a member may remain on the TDRL from five years to three years.
2017	• Department of Defense, Under Secretary of Defense, "Memorandum: Clarifying Guidance to Military Discharge Review Boards and Boards for Correction of Military/Naval Records Considering Requests by Veterans for Modifications of Their Discharge Due to Mental Health Conditions, Sexual Assault, or Sexual Harassment," was published.
2018	• Changes were incorporated into DoDI 1332.18, *Disability Evaluation System*, to include stricter guidelines for those wishing to go through the LDES.

we're going to fix it" (Baker, 2007). Shortly after this visit, President Bush issued an executive order to form the President's Commission on Care for America's Wounded Warriors and the Task Force on Returning Global War Heroes.

This commission, commonly called the Dole-Shalala Commission after its two chairs (President's Commission, 2007, p. 18), was required to examine post-deployment transitions for returning wounded service members, as well as the coordination and delivery of health care, disability, and other benefits. In the final report, the commission detailed the delays service members faced when being evaluated for disability adjudication and their dissatisfaction with and confusion regarding the system.[4] The commission recommended an overhaul of DES, empha-

---

[4]   The report also contained the findings from a survey of service members who had been medically evacuated from Iraq or Afghanistan. Less than 40 percent of respondents expressed

sizing the need for continuity of care and the elimination of the dual adjudication by DoD and VA. Specifically it recommended that DoD and VA should create a single, comprehensive, standardized medical examination. DoD would determine fitness, and VA would determine initial disability level. It also recommended that DoD and VA work to ensure the rapid transfer of patient information. Additionally, the report urged Congress to strengthen its efforts to help veterans with PTSD and TBI and suggested that "Congress should enable all veterans who have been deployed in Afghanistan and Iraq who need PTSD care to receive it from the VA" (President's Commission, 2007, p. 9).

In making its recommendations, the commission built on the findings of the President's Task Force on Returning Global War on Terror Heroes which were published earlier in 2007. The Task Force was chaired by VA Secretary Jim Nicholson. This task force had been charged with examining federal services available to service members returning from Iraq and Afghanistan and to issue a report within 45 days that identified gaps in those services and an action plan to ensure that federal agencies that support returning troops interact and cooperate effectively. The task force made 25 recommendations, including the recommendation for a single DoD/VA process for disability benefits determinations, development of a system of co-management to ease the transition from DoD to VA, expansion of VA access to DoD records to improve transfer of care, TBI screenings for all service members returning from Operation Enduring Freedom (OEF) and Operation Iraqi Freedom (OIF), and the creation of a database to track patients who have experienced TBI (VA, 2007).

In addition to the president's initiatives, a number of other commissions and task forces were working to investigate and address the concerns about the treatment of returning wounded service members. Several of the reports issuing from this work were influential in spurring changes to the disability evaluation process.

---

satisfaction with the system, and slightly more than 40 percent understood the evaluation system. Furthermore, approximately 40 percent of respondents took 21 weeks or more to complete the VA evaluation process. This meant a significant portion of the population waited seven months for VA payments and care at a VA facility.

- Defense Secretary Robert M. Gates created an Independent Review Group, also known as the Marsh-West Group,[5] in response to public criticism about the events at Walter Reed. The Marsh-West Group was tasked with reviewing the care and administrative processes at Walter Reed and the National Naval Medical Center in Bethesda, Maryland. Among other findings, the group reported in April 2007 that medical care was lacking for those suffering from TBI, PTSD, and other mental and behavioral health problems and that previous recommendations to make DES less confusing had been ignored. The report recommended the establishment of a center of excellence on the treatment of PTSD and TBI and an overhaul of DES (Independent Review Group, 2007).
- The Veterans Disability Benefits Commission was established by the 2004 NDAA to study the benefits provided to compensate and assist veterans for disabilities attributable to military service. In its final report, issued in August 2007, the Veterans Disability Benefits Commission found that the current rating system was confusing even to raters in some categories. The commission also found that VA ratings for individual conditions tended to be higher than DoD ratings for those conditions and that overall VA rated more conditions per veteran than DoD (Christensen et al., 2007).
- As part of its work, the Veterans Disability Benefits Commission was required to consult with IOM, which produced a separate report. This report recommended changes to VASRD, including a recommendation that it compensate not only for lost earnings but also for nonwork disability and loss of quality of life (McGeary et al., 2007).

To provide oversight and coordination of efforts to implement recommendations emanating from the various commissions and groups examining wounded warrior issues, the Secretaries of Veterans Affairs and Defense established the Wounded, Ill and Injured Senior

---

[5] The DoD Independent Review Group was chaired by John Marsh, a former member of Congress and former Army Secretary, and Togo West, also a former Army Secretary who subsequently served as the Secretary of VA.

Oversight Committee (SOC) in 2007. The SOC created eight lines of action (LOAs): (1) DES; (2) prevention, identification, treatment, recovery, rehabilitation, and research on TBI and PTSD; (3) case and care management; (4) the sharing of data between the two departments; (5) improving medical facilities; (6) designing a continuous care plan; (7) reviewing and coordinating the latest legislation related to wounded warriors and their families; and (8) personnel, pay, and financial support (VA and DoD, 2009, p. 3).

In July 2007, Congress passed the Dignified Treatment of Wounded Warriors Act (S. 1606, July 25, 2007), which included provisions to evaluate and alter the disability system. Language from this bill regarding the disability evaluation process and transition out of the military was ultimately included in the 2008 NDAA (Pub. L. 110-181, Sub. A, §1643, 2008; Simmons, 2015, p. 61).[6]

2008 National Defense Authorization Act: Big Changes to the Disability Evaluation System

The 2008 NDAA established major changes to DES and laid the groundwork for a transition to IDES. The changes required by NDAA were intended to address the numerous recommendations to improve the DES and transition process for returning wounded service members. In particular, NDAA required DoD to pilot a joint DoD-VA disability evaluation process, improve consistency between the departments, improve the timeliness of the disability evaluation process, and increase service members' opportunities to appeal. We discuss each of these changes below.

2008 National Defense Authorization Act Disability Evaluation System Pilot Program

The 2008 NDAA authorized the establishment of pilot programs to explore different ways to conduct DoD and VA disability ratings. In the end, only one pilot was conducted; in it, the VA conducted the dis-

---

[6] Congressional staff indicated that the language for disability system improvements was included in the NDAA because they knew the bill would pass, something that was not assured as a stand-alone piece of legislation.

ability examinations and assigned VASRDs, while DoD made the final disability determination. The goal of this pilot was to reduce processing times under DES, eliminate or alter unnecessary or harmful applicable statutes or regulations, and eliminate variation between the military branches (Pub. L. 110-181, Sub. A, §1644, 2008). The pilot would eventually become IPDES and then later IDES (Simmons, 2015, p. 58).[7]

Changes to Improve Disability Rating Consistency

The 2008 NDAA called for DoD and VA to jointly "develop and implement a policy on improvements to the care, management and transition of recovering service members" (Pub. L. 110-181, Sub. A, §1611, 2008) and required a feasibility assessment of consolidating VA and DoD DESs as part of that goal to increase consistency of ratings between the DoD and VA (Pub. L. 110-181, Sub. A, §1612, 2008). It also called for secretaries of both departments to implement uniform processes and procedures.[8] As part of this effort to increase consistency, the law mandated that DoD use VASRD for assigning disability ratings. Although the law allowed DoD and VA to jointly select different rating criteria, they were only permitted to do so only if the new criteria would result in a higher disability rating.

In implementing the law, DoD issued new policy guidance, stating that military departments (e.g., Army, Navy) could not deviate

---

[7] Congressional staff interviewed about this pilot indicated that it was a major shift by the military to cede control of disability determination to VA and to use the VASRD. This change had been discussed before, but the situation had become sufficiently urgent due to the media attention surrounding the Walter Reed incident that it was finally accomplished.

[8] Relevant instruction in Public Law 110-181, Public Law 110-181, National Defense Authorization Act for Fiscal Year 2008 Sub. A, §1614: Transition of Recovering Service Members from Care and Treatment Through DoD to Through VA, January 28, 2008, concerns

- procedures for identifying and tracking service members during transition
- procedures and timelines for enrolling recovering service members in applicable VA systems
- procedures for the transmittal of records and other information from DoD to VA
- a process for the use of joint separation and evaluation physical examination that meets both DoD and VA requirements.

from VASRD or any interpretation of VASRD, except in unusual cases (DoD OUSD[P&R], 2008).[9, 10]

The policy change to require the consistent use of VASRD had a particular impact on service members with conditions for which the previous DoD rating guidance differed significantly from a strict application of VASRD. Two conditions serve as exemplars: PTSD and sleep apnea. For PTSD (and indeed, all mental health conditions), DoD had previously assessed severity based on the extent of "loss of function . . . reflected in impaired social and industrial adaptability" (DoDI 1332.39, 1996); ratings were based on functional impairment related to competence, presence of psychosis, hospitalization status, need for supervision, job stability, social adjustment, need for medications and psychotherapy, and risk of harm to self and others. In contrast, the new policy required that service members who were determined to be unfit because of "mental disorders due to traumatic stress" (e.g., PTSD) were to receive a *minimum 50 percent disability rating* and be placed on TDRL and reevaluated within six months (unless their total disability rating was 80 percent or higher, in which case they should be permanently retired) (38 CFR. § 4.129, 1996). For sleep apnea, previous rating guidance was based on "civilian earning capacity," whereby service members with "total industrial impairment" were rated at 100 percent, and those with "mild industrial impairment" were rated at 0 percent. The new policy required the strict application of VASRD, for which ratings are based on clinical criteria—for example, if sleep apnea causes a service member to not feel rested after sleeping, it is rated at 30 percent, and if the service member uses a breathing machine, such as a continuous positive airway pressure machine, during sleep, it is rated at 50 percent.

---

[9]   Department of Defense, Office of the Under Secretary of Defense (Personnel and Readiness) Policy Memorandum on "Implementing Disability-Related Provisions of the National Defense Authorization Act of 2008 (Pub. L. 110-181)," October 14, 2008, rescinded DoDI 1332.39 and directed military departments to use only the VASRD ratings. In addition, DoDI 1332.38 was updated with policy from the now-rescinded DoDI 1332.39.

[10]   Note that U.S. Code, Title 10, Section 1216a simply states that the military departments will abide by VASRD to the extent feasible but may rely on criteria jointly prescribed by the Secretaries of VA and DoD.

Changes to Improve Timeliness

To address concerns that the disability evaluation process took too long, timeline goals were established for each step in the disability process. DoD implemented these requirements in a policy memorandum (DoD, October 14, 2008, pp. 3–6) altering an existing DoDI (DoDI 1332.38, 1996) in accordance with this section of the law and ensured that timeliness and caseload standards applied to all service members in the DES.

The policy memorandum also made several changes to DES operational standards, including adding various timeline standards for both service members and military departments. However, some elements of this timeline standard created reporting ambiguities, such as the fact that the service member transition phase, ostensibly 45 days, did not include any administrative absences they were authorized to take (DoDM 1332.18, 2014b, p. 40).

Changes to Increase Ability to Appeal

The 2008 NDAA also altered the procedures for service members' review of their disability determinations. Under guidance issued by DoD, service members could request a review by an impartial health care professional of the medical evidence included in the MEB findings (DoD, October 14, 2008, p. 2). The impartial health care professional could advise on whether the findings were accurate, and the service member could then request a review based on the advice. The results of the impartial medical review were to be forwarded to the MEB "as required" (DoD, 2011, p. 20).

Finally, responding to evidence of disparities in disability ratings across the military departments under LDES, and the new requirements for strict and consistent application of VASRD, the 2008 NDAA also created PDBR to review PEB disability determinations for individuals who were medically separated with a disability rating of 20 percent disability or less and who were therefore not eligible for retirement (Pub. L. 110-181, Sub. A, § 1643, 2008). DoD issued DoDI 6040.44 to implement PDBR, clarifying that PDBR was to review disability ratings only, not the determinations of fitness. PDBR could make recommendations to the secretary of the service branch from which the service member was discharged to re-characterize separation or modify the rating, recharacterize separation to retirement for disability, or modify the rating upward (DoDI 6040.44, 2008, pp. 9–10). The rating was not to be lowered, however. This DoDI, consistent with the law, limited PDBR eligibility to those individuals who were separated between September 11, 2001, and December 31, 2009. In 2009, the policy was altered slightly to increase PDBR's scope, stating that "the PDBR may, at the request of an eligible member . . . review conditions identified but not determined to be unfitting by the PEB" (DoDI 6040.44, 2008). This DoDI explained that PDBR was entitled to recommend that a finding of fitness be changed to unfitness and assign a rating to the condition (DoDI 6040.44, 2008). Once the PDBR was created, all eligible service members (approximately 73,000) were contacted and informed of their eligibility for a case review. Of these, about 18,000 had submitted applications for review as of December 2017.[11] After review, 18 percent had their disposition changed from medical separation to medical retirement (increased total disability rating to 30 percent or greater), 25 percent had an increase in their medical separation rating (but no change to disposition), and about half (56 percent) had no change (PDBR, 2017).

2009–2010: Introduction of the Integrated Pilot Disability Evaluation System

The pilot projects to examine the feasibility of creating a single, integrated DoD/VA DES were first initiated in 2007 at the direction of SOC (LOA-1) at three national capital region sites: Walter Reed Army Medical Center, National Naval Medical Center-Bethesda, and Andrews Air Force Base. In November 2008, DoD and VA entered into an MOA to establish the scope, policy, responsibilities, and implementing instructions for the DES Pilot (DoD, 2008). It included the DES Pilot Operations Manual, which provided guidance for the main element of the pilot: a single disability medical examination and a "single-sourced rating system" (DoD, November 2008).

---

[11] Physical Disability Board of Review, personal communication with authors, December 2017.

In June 2009, DoD and VA entered into an MOA to expand these pilot sites, and by 2010, 24 sites had been added to the pilot (GAO, 2010b, p. 1; GAO, 2012),[12] which then became known as the Integrated Pilot Disability Evaluation System (IPDES) (VA and DoD, 2009).

For those cases referred into IPDES, DoD and VA agreed on a few key elements:

1. "The medical examination will include a complete review of systems and a comprehensive evaluation of medical conditions identified and referred to the IPDES by a military medical provider" (VA and DoD, 2009, Sec. 4.A) as well as other conditions claimed by the service member. Examiners were directed to use the VA Compensation & Pension (C&P) General Medical examination worksheet and applicable VA Automated Medical Information Exchange examination worksheets to the extent feasible.
2. VA had the choice to provide the disability examination. If VA declined, then DoD would perform it.
3. VA would provide VA C&P disability examination training and certification to individuals both ordering and performing examinations.
4. Whether VA or the military department performed the disability examination, both would provide the results to each other, to DoD for fitness determinations and dispositions of unfit service members, and to VA for disability ratings (VA and DoD, 2009, pp. 3–4). Confirming prior practice, ratings were completed using VASRD. The IPDES MOA made clear that having a single rating agency was a major goal (VA and DoD, 2009, p. 5).

Figure 2.1 demonstrates IDES, when it was in the IPDES phase, as compared with the legacy process.

In 2010, GAO found that the average time a service member waited for adjudication had been cut almost in half under IPDES as

---

[12] MOA noted that the sites were the military treatment facilities (MTFs) included in the September 25, 2008, OUSD (P&R) memorandum, subject to further expansion.

Figure 2.1
Legacy Disability Evaluation Compared with the Pilot of the Integrated Disability Evaluation System Process

Legacy process

Actions performed by Department of Defense (DoD)

1. Service member referred to disability system.

2. Military medical providers conduct medical exam.

3. Medical evaluation board (MEB) identifies conditions that may make member unfit for duty.

4. Physical evaluation board (PEB) assesses service member's fitness for duty.

5. If found unfit, PEB rates the unfitting conditions to determine benefits.

6. Service member discharged with DoD benefits if eligible.

Actions performed by Veterans Affairs (VA)

  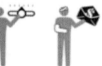

7. Veteran files claim for benefits with VA.

8. VA providers examine veteran.

9. VA rates all of vet's service-connected conditions.

10. Veteran receives VA benefits if eligible.

Integrated Disability Evaluation System process

Actions performed by DoD and VA

1. Service member referred to disability system.

2. Medical providers conduct medical exam to VA standards.

3. Medical evaluation board (MEB) identifies conditions that may make member unfit for duty.

4. Physical evaluation board (PEB) assesses service member's fitness for duty.

5. If found unfit, VA rates the conditions to determine both DoD and VA benefits.

6. Service member receives both DoD and VA benefits shortly after discharge.

SOURCE: GAO, 2010a, p. 5.

compared with DES. Furthermore, satisfaction reported by service members was higher under IPDES than under LDES. However, GAO also reported that there were staffing and logistical challenges that needed to be addressed prior to the full rollout of IDES (GAO, 2010a, pp. 7–10).

Finally, during this same time period, DoD issued a policy memorandum allowing military departments to expedite service members through DES in certain cases, such as when a service member had experienced a catastrophic injury (Military Health System, undated[a]). This did not impact the transition from LDES to IDES, but rather constituted a new change to DES. The memorandum revised DoDI 1332.38, *Disability Evaluation System*, by adding that a service member's condition may be designated catastrophic, and the service member may then waive DES evaluation and be rated with a 100 percent combined disability rating. This process is known as expedited DES (EDES) (DoD, 2009, p. 1).

2011: Integrated Disability Evaluation System Implementation

After the success of IPDES, DoD and VA formally established IDES in 2011 (DoD, 2011).[13] The key element of IDES, as described by the official policy, was consistent with the goals set forth in the pilot phase: "a single set of disability medical examinations appropriate for fitness determination by the Military Departments and a single set of disability ratings provided by VA for appropriate use by both departments" (DoD, 2011, p. 10).

Under IDES, the disability evaluation process now includes the following steps:

1. The service member enters IDES upon referral from a military care provider because an injury or illness makes it difficult for the service member to perform his or her duties consistent with his or her office, grade, rank, or rating. The military care provider also gives the referral to a military treatment facility

---

[13] The new policy was incorporated into DoDI 1332.38 and canceled the various DTMs that had been promulgated regarding the DES pilots.

(MTF) patient administrator, who assigns a PEBLO to the service member.

2. A VA medical examiner performs an examination.[14] The case file, which includes the results of the medical examinations, is provided to the MEB convening authority, which consists of two to three medical officers appointed by the local MTF. MEB determines if the service member will make a full recovery and if it is decided that he or she will, the service member is placed on temporary limited duty.[15] Otherwise, the service member is referred to the informal PEB (IPEB) (DoDI 1332.18).

3. If IPEB finds the service member to be unfit for duty, they request the proposed disability ratings be prepared by the VA Disability Evaluation System Rating Activity Site (D-RAS), and then, upon receipt, provide its findings to the service member. The service member may request a formal PEB (FPEB) if he or she disagrees with the findings of IPEB. If requested, FPEB adjudicates the case and provides its findings to the service member.

4. The service member may then appeal the FPEB findings. The military department considers the appeal, and then the service member is either returned to duty, separated, medically retired, or transferred to another service.

5. As part of this, prior to release, the service member needs to also file "claim for compensation, pension, or hospitalization" to VA or sign a statement that he or she has refused to file a claim. This is not a new policy, but it is required in IDES (10 U.S.C. §1218, 2008).

6. If the service member is separated or medically retired for disability through IDES, the military department and VA provide disability compensation and benefits. If a service member

---

[14] During this phase, a VA Medical Service Coordinator works with the service member to prepare a claim for VA benefits.

[15] Placement on permanent limited duty, with a profile of either P3 or P4, as the result of having a condition that does not appear to meet medical retention standards, is often what triggers a soldier's referral to IDES. See DoDI 1332.18.

is placed on TDRL, the military department will periodically reexamine and readjudicate the case (DoD, 2011, pp. 10–11).

The 2011 policy also provided timeliness goals. For active component service members, the stated goal was no more than 295 days from referral to either return to duty or disability discharge and notification of the VA benefits decision. The MEB phase should take no more than 100 days; the PEB phase, 120 days; the transition phase, 45 days; and finally, the VA disability compensation phase, 30 days.

2011–2018: Evolution of the Integrated Disability Evaluation System

Since the implementation of IDES in 2011, there have been several significant changes, including (1) renewed use of the legacy system, (2) increased attention paid to administrative separations, (3) reductions in TDRL, and (4) more stringent timeliness standards.

Reintroduction of the Legacy Disability Evaluation System

The policy (DTM 11-015) that introduced IDES in 2011 had explained that "IDES . . . is superseding the legacy Disability Evaluation System (DES)" (DoD, 2011, p. 1). However, due to a 2015 policy memorandum, LDES was not completely canceled (DoD, 2015). The policy memorandum stated that, if requested by a service member, the secretaries of the military departments could authorize processing through LDES rather than IDES. The memo also explained that Secretaries could direct a member for processing through LDES if going through IDES would detrimentally impact the member or the service (DoD, 2015). According to disability policy experts we spoke with, the option to be evaluated under the legacy system was introduced to allow service members who were injured during initial training to be processed out of the military quickly rather than spending nearly a year in IDES. While initially designed for trainees and other groups of service members, under the revised policy any service member could be processed through LDES. Requests were typically made by the DES convening authority, the service member, or the service member's commanding officer, and decisions are handled on a case-by-case basis. Unlike in IDES, only DoD is involved in legacy cases; DoD conducts the medical exam and the ratings. The service member then has the option of filing a claim with VA separately, after discharge. Along with the updated DoDI, DoD also published a lengthy manual about DESs, with Volume 1 focusing on LDES, and Volume 2 on IDES (DoDM 1332.18, 2014a, 2014b).

In 2018, the policy was revised again to limit the use of LDES. The revised policy made clear that "it is DoD policy for service members to process through the IDES unless a compelling and individualized reason for process through the LDES is approved by the Secretary of the Military Department" (DoDI 1332.18, 2018, p. 2). In the enclosure outlining procedure, DoDI explains that the secretaries of the military departments are to use IDES for "all newly initiated cases referred under the duty related process" except for those approved for the LDES. For all other new cases, the secretaries may authorize processing for service members, including recruits, trainees, and midshipmen, processing under LDES after providing the member a legal briefing on the procedural differences between IDES and LDES; enroll the member in LDES if they had provided the member with information about VA Benefits Delivery at Discharge program before enrollment; or use LDES for consenting members designated with a catastrophic illness or injury incurred in the line of duty (DoDI 1332.18, 2018, Enclosure 3, pp. 15–16). The 2018 DoDI also completely eliminated the use of EDES (DoDI 1332.18, 2018, p. 1).

Administrative Separations

An administrative separation is an involuntary separation from the military (akin to being "fired") for reasons of misconduct, poor performance, alcohol or drug use problems, having a physical or mental condition that impacts performance but does not meet criteria for disability, or other reasons. Service members who are separated through this process may have different discharge characterizations, depending on the circumstances: honorable; general (under honorable conditions); other than honorable conditions; or dishonorable. Service members may not qualify for VA or other benefits if they have an unfavorable discharge characterization, although recent policy changes have been implemented to ensure access to VA mental health care for veterans with unfavorable discharges (sometimes known as "bad paper" discharges) (H.R. 1685, 2017).

Although most service members with serious mental or physical health conditions are referred to DES, there was concern that some service members were being administratively separated for misconduct due to consequences of their mental health problems (Emery, 2006). The 2010 NDAA required that the service branches assess the impact of a PTSD or TBI diagnosis on service members prior to discharging them for misconduct, and subsequent DoD policy changes were made in response (Pub. L. 111-84, 2009; DTM 10-022, 2010; DoDI 1332.14, 2014). In 2014, updated DoD policy (DoDI 1332.14) required that enlisted service members who are undergoing administrative separations be evaluated for PTSD or TBI to determine if there are extenuating circumstances for the separation including whether the member was deployed overseas or was sexually assaulted in the prior two years; is being administratively separated under a characterization that is not general or honorable; has been either diagnosed with PTSD or TBI or reasonably alleges PTSD or TBI based on deployment to a contingency or sexual assault in the previous two years; and is not being separated due to a court martial or other UCMJ proceeding (DoDI 1332.14, 2014, p. 49). The 2015 NDAA required an investigation into the impact of mental and physical trauma on misconduct discharges (Pub. L. 113-291, 2014), and a subsequent GAO report found that service branches were inconsistently screening service members for PTSD and TBI prior to administrative separation (GAO, 2017).

Service branches were also required to review previous administrative separation discharges to consider whether PTSD or TBI could have been a factor. In 2017, DoD issued a memorandum that directed the military departments' boards for discharge review and correction of records to liberalize the considerations for discharge relief, meaning it was easier to appeal the decision for a less than honorable discharge for service members who had been separated due to mental health conditions (DoD, 2017). We discuss this in greater detail in the next chapter.

Temporary Disability Retired List and Timeliness Standards

The 2017 NDAA amended U.S. Code, Title 10, Section 1210, reducing the maximum time a member may remain on the TDRL from five years to three years (Pub. L. 114-328, 2016). This was incorporated into the revised DoDI 1332.18, effective in 2018 (DoDI 1332.18, 2018, Appendix 4 to Enclosure 3, p. 46). This change was made because a DoD study found that the overwhelming majority of service members who were on TDRL for more than three years were permanently retired (DoD, Office of the Under Secretary of Defense [Personnel and Readiness], undated). This report, as well as an earlier GAO report that investigated the temporary retirement process, recommended the change from five to three years (GAO, 2009a).

More recently, timeliness standards for IDES have been under review. At the time of this report, policy recommendations had been introduced to reduce the timeliness goal to 180 days,[16] a significant decrease from the 295-day goal when IDES was first implemented in 2011 and from the timeliness goal of 230 days established in 2018 (DTM-18-004, 2018).

---

[16] Office of the Secretary of Defense, Health Affairs, personal communication with authors, 2019. The 180-day timeliness goal was established later in 2019 through DTM-18-004, Change 2.

CHAPTER THREE

Posttraumatic Stress Disorder and Traumatic Brain Injury: Signature Injuries of the Wars in Iraq and Afghanistan

As noted in the previous chapter, attention to the needs of returning service members resulted not only in major changes to DES, but also in significant changes to the recognition and treatment of the signature injuries of the wars in Iraq and Afghanistan: PTSD and TBI. DoD policy changes and new initiatives related to awareness, screening, and treatment of PTSD and TBI in the military health system significantly altered the landscape for service members who experienced these wounds. In this chapter, we provide some context for the attention to PTSD and TBI and focus specifically on how DoD policies around screening for these conditions among service members evolved over time. We also describe how the growing recognition and understanding of PTSD and TBI led to changes in DES policies for these conditions.

Background

As early as 2003 there was increased focus on the psychological toll of the wars in Iraq and Afghanistan on returning service members. For example, when the U.S. Army Surgeon General chartered the Mental Health Advisory Team (MHAT) in 2003 to assess mental health issues related to Iraq combat deployments, it found higher than historical suicide rates, high levels of stress, low morale, and low rates of treatment seeking (*OIF MHAT,* 2003). In subsequent years, MHAT documented continued behavioral health needs among deployed soldiers in Iraq and Afghanistan and provided recommendations for improving the delivery of behavioral health care to these soldiers. A 2004 GAO report suggested that VA should prepare for 15 percent of service members returning from Iraq and Afghanistan to have PTSD and noted that early identification and treatment would be essential (GAO, 2004a). Media reports around this time also highlighted the mental health needs of returning service members, noting high rates of suicide, depression, and PTSD (Carey, 2005).

Responding to the increasing awareness of the mental health needs of returning service members, the 2006 NDAA required the formation of a DoD Task Force on Mental Health to "examine matters relating to mental health and the Armed Forces." The task force produced 95 recommendations for improvements to the mental health of service members and their families (DoD, Task Force on Mental Health, 2007), including recommendations to build a culture of support for psychological health, ensure the delivery of high-quality behavioral health care for service members and their families, and provide adequate resources for behavioral health care. The presidential and DoD commissions mentioned in the previous chapter, which were tasked with investigating the care for service members with combat-related conditions, produced findings with a similar recommendation that additional attention and resources needed to be devoted to the detection and treatment of TBI, PTSD, and other mental health issues (Christensen et al., 2007; Independent Review Group, 2007; President's Commission, 2007; Task Force on Returning Global War on Terror Heroes, 2007).

Around the same time, studies of service members who deployed in support of the Iraq and Afghanistan wars highlighted an increased prevalence of PTSD and TBI among this population. Seminal publications in the *Journal of the American Medical Association* and the *New England Journal of Medicine* revealed that deployment to these operations may be associated with higher risk for PTSD among soldiers and marines (Milliken, Auchterlonie, and Hoge, 2007; Hoge et al., 2008). That these studies were conducted by military researchers reflected

DoD's investment in better understanding these important issues. A 2008 RAND study on *Invisible Wounds of War: Psychological and Cognitive Injuries, Their Consequences, and Services to Assist Recovery* highlighted the high rates of PTSD and TBI among all returning service members and the low frequency with which these individuals received high-quality care (Tanielian and Jaycox, 2008).

IOM also conducted a number of studies during this time to describe the impact of combat on mental health and make recommendations for addressing the mental health needs of service members and veterans.[1] In 2006–2007, VA commissioned IOM to examine the diagnosis, assessment, treatment, and compensation of PTSD for veterans (IOM, 2006, 2007a, 2007b). The resulting reports documented the current state of the science for PTSD diagnosis and treatment and made recommendations for changes to how VA evaluated disability due to PTSD. In particular, the IOM reports recommended the establishment of new VASRD criteria for PTSD based on consistent diagnostic standards and a fixed long-term minimum level of disability benefit for veterans with service-connected PTSD. Congress included a provision in the 2010 NDAA for the commission of another IOM study to assess PTSD care in the military and VA. The resulting reports found that while both departments had made substantial investments in the treatment of PTSD, there was a lack of standards for reporting and evaluation—for example, neither department was consistently providing evidence-based treatments for PTSD (IOM, 2014).

In 2012, President Obama issued an Executive order aimed at improving mental health care for wounded warriors (Obama, 2012). Among other requirements, the Executive order established an interagency task force and required a national research action plan to address diagnosis and treatment of PTSD, TBI, and suicide. In a 2013 report, the Congressional Research Service recommended that Congress monitor research on the physical manifestations of psychological health conditions, the effectiveness of screening and treatment efforts, service member access to mental health care, the quality of mental

---

[1]   IOM was renamed the Health and Medicine Division of the National Academies of Sciences, Engineering, and Medicine in March 2016.

health care, ongoing programming, and the costs of current and future mental health care. The report specified that a better understanding of this research would put Congress in a better position to consider implications for policy and understanding of gaps in research (Blakeley and Jansen, 2013).

As attention to and awareness of the needs of returning service members grew with regard to these signature injuries, and in response to recommendations from the DoD Task Force on Mental Health, DoD made significant changes to how it organized psychological health resources and capabilities (DoD, Task Force on Mental Health, 2007). One major outcome was the creation of the Defense Centers of Excellence (DCoE) for Psychological Health and Traumatic Brain Injury. DCoE aimed "to assess, validate, oversee and facilitate prevention, resilience, identification, treatment, outreach, rehabilitation, and reintegration programs for PH and TBI to ensure DoD meets the needs of service members, veterans, military families, and communities" (DoD, 2009). To carry this out, DCoE partnered with DoD, VA, and a national network of military and civilian agencies, clinical experts, advocacy groups, and academic institutions to establish best practices and quality standards for addressing psychological health including TBI.[2]

In addition, DoD implemented other major changes in response to recommendations from the DoD Task Force on Mental Health, including the creation of the position of director of psychological health within each military department, leadership training to promote prevention and treatment, and a campaign to reduce stigma around mental health treatment. DoD also made changes to mental health staffing to increase the availability of mental health treatment, including integrating mental health into primary care settings, and to improve access. Finally, DoD prioritized providing evidence-based treatments, monitoring the quality of care, and attending to transitions between care settings, and at the same time invested in research and program evaluation to ensure service members benefited from high-quality care (Acosta et al., 2014b; Martin et al., 2014; Ryan et al., 2014).

---

[2] In 2017, DCoE for Psychological Health and Traumatic Brain Injury was reorganized into separate centers within the Defense Health Agency.

In the next sections, we will further detail DoD policy changes related to screening to identify individuals with PTSD or TBI and policy changes relevant to these conditions related to disability evaluation. DoD's educational efforts and programs designed to reduce the stigma associated with mental health within the military have been previously reviewed (Seal et al., 2007; Weinick et al., 2011; Acosta et al., 2014a), and treatment of PTSD and TBI has also been covered in other research (Hoge et al., 2004; Hoge, Auchterlonie, and Milliken, 2006; Acosta et al., 2014b; Acosta et al., 2018; Farmer et al., 2016; Hepner et al., 2017a, 2017b; Tanielian et al., 2008).

Policy Changes to Increase Screening for Posttraumatic Stress Disorder and Traumatic Brain Injury

Routine screening for physical and mental health problems allows for early identification, treatment, and, with effective interventions, recovery. Screening also allows for population surveillance and the appropriate allocation of resources. In the military context, screening for combat-related conditions can be used to identify service members potentially in need of care, make referrals to appropriate care when warranted, and alleviate or minimize ongoing health problems. If a treating provider determines that the service member is unlikely to return to full duty, he or she may refer the patient for disability evaluation. Changes to screening policies and practices may have a downstream effect on the number and characteristics of service members who receive diagnoses, treatment, and referral to DES. In fact, a 2018 analysis found that changes to DoD TBI screening policies were associated with a 78–124 percent increase in reporting, depending on screening tool and service (Agimi et al., 2018).

The military conducts several regular screenings for mental health problems and TBI. The most significant of these with regard to disability and medical retirement processes are the Pre- and Post-Deployment Health Assessments (Pre-DHA, PDHA), the Post-Deployment Health Re-Assessment (PDHRA), and the Mental Health Assessment (MHA). Below, we describe these screening tools, along with their origins and significant policy changes that occurred since 2001.

Deployment Health Assessments

Currently, service members deploying to a theater of combat are required to complete a Pre-DHA within 120 days prior to deployment and a PDHA within 30 days of returning from the deployment, forms Defense Department (DD) 2795 and DD 2796, respectively. This is the way the assessments are supposed to work, but they are not always consistently applied. The assessments contain questions relating to physical and mental health as well as potential environmental exposures and relationship stressors (DoD, DD Form 2795, 2012; DoD, DD Form 2796, 2015). Beginning in 2006, service members were also required to have a face-to-face interview during in-theater medical out-processing or within 30 days of returning home to discuss their responses to the PDHA and any concerns they may have about their health or exposures during deployment.[3] Individuals who indicate health concerns are to be referred for a meeting with a trained health care provider (DoDI 6490.03, 2011, pp. 28–29). Finally, service members who complete a PDHA are also expected to complete a PDHRA (DoD, DD Form 2900, 2005) between 90 and 180 days of their return home from deployment; this is intended to identify physical or mental health problems that emerge after completion of the PDHA (ASD[HA], 2005a). After completion of the PDHRA, a health care provider is to discuss health concerns with the service member, educate the service member on post-deployment health readjustment issues, provide information on resources available for assistance (DoDI 6490.03, 2011, p. 31) and make any necessary referrals. These assessments are to be conducted for every service member who deploys, and, although the records from these assessments could be considered in the IDES process as they are part of the medical record, they do not constitute a disability evaluation.

The predecessor to the PDHA was established in 1997 in response to concerns about Gulf War Syndrome believed to be associated with deployment to Operation Desert Storm (DoDI 6490.2, 1997; DoDI 6490.3, 1997). Later that year, as part of the 1998 NDAA, the PDHA

---

[3] The requirement to conduct face-to-face interviews was specified in 2006 in DoDI 6490.03, *Deployment Health.*

was established and codified into law (Pub. L. 105-85, 1997; 10 U.S.C. §1074f, 2012). The law required a surveillance system to include (a) a pre-deployment medical examination, (b) a post-deployment medical examination, and (c) record-keeping for fiscal year 1999 and the next five consecutive years (Pub. L. 105-85, 1997; 10 U.S.C. §1074f, 2012). As a result of this policy change, forms DD 2795 and DD 2796 were created to track this information. However, there have been subsequent reports that question the compliance and consistency of implementation of the screening tools across the service branches (Curtain, 2003; GAO, 2004b).

The PDHRA was established in September 2006 (DoDI 6490.03, 2011, p. 31) following a 2005 memorandum from the Assistant Secretary of Defense for Health Affairs (ASD[HA]). This memo explained the need for such a reassessment because many service members developed physical or mental health problems months after the PDHA had been completed (ASD[HA], 2005a). A 2004 study by Army researchers had first identified delayed onset of these post-deployment issues (Bliese et al., 2004; Hoge et al., 2004; GAO, 2008). In 2011, U.S. Code 10 §1074f was amended to codify the PDHRA into law (Pub. L. 111-383, Div. A, Title VII, 2011). Per the legislation, the reassessment was specifically designed to "identify health concerns, including mental health concerns, that may become manifest several months following their deployment" (Pub. L. 111-383, Div. A, Title VII, 2011). The legislation also codified the time frames for the separate assessments to be conducted.

The PDHA and PDHRA screen for PTSD using the four-item Primary Care PTSD Screen (PC-PTSD) (Prins et al., 2003). While use of this tool has not changed over time, between 2005 and 2011, the PDHA and PDHRA were revised to include enhanced mental health screening tools and a mild TBI screening tool (Pub. L. 109–364, 2006). In 2008, the PDHA was revised to include TBI screening measures, which had been required by the 2007 NDAA (Pub. L. 109–364, 2006). Since then, the PDHA has included a four-item tool to assess mild TBI. Although there have been some concerns about the validity of this tool (Hoge, Goldberg, and Castro, 2009)—and, more broadly, DoD's definition of mild TBI—the tool itself has remained in the PDHA, albeit with some slight alteration in 2012 to collect even more detailed information about the specifics of the head injury (e.g., duration of loss of consciousness).

In 2008, after a GAO report found low completion rates for the PDHAs (GAO, 2008b), DoD required that DD Forms 2766, 2795, and 2796 be integrated into the service member's permanent medical health records within 30 days of their return to a demobilization site or their home station (DoDI 6490.03, 2011, p. 30; GAO, 2008b). That same year, GAO also studied the implementation of the new mental health portions of the PDHA and PDHRA. It found that while DoD had taken steps to implement the new screening standards, health care providers had limited ability to track whether service members who screened positive for mental health problems completed a referral for mental health care (GAO, 2008a). A separate GAO report found that DoD was unable to accurately assess whether service members completed the PDHRA because of limitations in the type and consistency of information available from the service branches (GAO, 2008b).

The following year, in 2009, another GAO report found that fewer than 80 percent of those who were required to do so had actually completed the PDHRA (GAO, 2009b). There have also been questions about the validity of the screening results themselves because service members may not be comfortable reporting mental health symptoms due to concerns about repercussions for their career or other factors. Research published in 2011 found that the PDHA may not accurately identify service members with PTSD. The study showed that reporting of PTSD symptoms, depression, suicidal ideation, and interest in receiving care was two to four times higher when screening was administered anonymously as compared with routine PDHA screening, which is tied to a service member's medical record. The study also found that 20 percent of soldiers who screened positive for PTSD or depression when the screening was anonymous reported that they had been uncomfortable answering the screening questions honestly on the PDHA, due to concerns about stigma about mental illness (Warner et al., 2011). While these assessment forms are still widely used, there are some questions about their ability to accurately identify all or even most service members with mental health problems, a common shortcoming of any self-report measure that relies on the veracity of self-report.

Mental Health Assessment

Since 2009, all deployed service members have been required to complete an MHA before and after each deployment. The MHA is an online, self-reported assessment that is followed by a face-to-face clinical interview. Per DoDI 6490.12, *Mental Health Assessments for Service Members Deployed in Connection with a Contingency Operation,* "The purpose of the deployment mental health assessment is to identify mental health conditions including posttraumatic stress disorder (PTSD), suicidal tendencies, and other behavioral health conditions that require referral for additional care and treatment in order to ensure individual and unit readiness" (DoDI 6490.12, 2013, p. 5).

The MHA was first mandated by Congress in the 2010 NDAA (Pub. L. 111-84, 2009). This legislation outlined the timing of the MHA, as well as how they should be administered (e.g., in a private setting, with personnel trained to administer such assessments, and so on). The law further required that the MHA be shared with VA, and that the assessments should cease when the service member leaves the military. In 2010 and 2011, some further clarification was provided by ASD(HA) (ASD[HA], 2010, 2011). The 2011 DTM officially established the policy (ASD[HA], 2011, p. 1). Since then, policies governing the timing and nature of the MHA have changed several times. The 2012 NDAA required DoD to implement regulations for the MHA, which included a standard set of assessment questions to be included on Pre-DHA and PDHA (Pub. L. 112-81, 2011).

The timeline of the MHA administration was altered in the 2013 NDAA, and official instruction on the changes was provided via a DoDI (Pub. L. 112-239, 2013; DoDI 6490.12, 2013). In the 2015 NDAA, the MHA was altered again so that every service member must complete an MHA every year and during deployments (Pub. L. 113-291, 2014). Most recently, the MHA has been included as part of service members' annual Periodic Health Assessment (DoDI 6200.06, 2016).

Currently, the MHA is supposed to be conducted for all service members who are deployed (with some narrow exceptions). It has four stages: 120 days or less prior to deployment (pre-deployment), once during each 180-day period a service member is deployed (during deployment), and then 181 days to 18 months (545 days), and 18 months (546 days) to 30 months (910 days) after return from deployment (post-deployment). In order to streamline the process, the first MHA is conducted in conjunction with the pre-DHA, and following deployment the MHA is administered in conjunction with the second PDHA and PDHRA. The final two MHA exams are conducted in conjunction with the service member's Periodic Health Assessment (Military Health System, undated[b]).[4] MHAs, including those administered in relation to a deployment and the annual assessment, are aligned so that each administration includes the same screening tool, which allows for consistency and tracking of service members' mental health over time.

The MHA screens for PTSD in three stages. The first is PC-PTSD, a five-item screening assessment for PTSD that was originally designed for use in primary care settings. If the service member has a positive screen on the PC-PTSD, the service member is supposed to complete the PTSD Checklist-Civilian version. This is a more detailed, 17-item measure that can be used to make a provisional diagnosis of PTSD (Weathers et al., 2013). If this screening is positive, a health care provider is to conduct a clinical interview with the service member. In the 2018 Report to Congress on MHAs (required by the 2015 NDAA), DoD recommended updating the MHA PTSD screening questions to align with the *Diagnostic and Statistical Manual of Mental Disorders* (DSM-5) (Office of the Secretary of Defense, 2018). As noted above, any changes to screening tools will likely have a downstream effect on the number of service members who are referred for mental health treatment, and potentially, the number who are referred to IDES.

Traumatic Brain Injury Screening

In addition to screening for mild TBI as part of the PDHA/PDHRA, DoD implemented additional TBI screening for service members on combat deployments to ensure that those who had experienced a TBI were adequately identified and treated. In 2006, the Defense and Veterans Brain Injury Center developed the Military Acute Concussion Evaluation (MACE) to evaluate TBI among service members who had

---

[4]   The Periodic Health Assessment is a screening tool that is used to evaluate the medical status of service members. It includes a self-reported health status, measurement and documentation of vitals (height, weight, and so on), review of current medical conditions, focused exam to identify conditions (as required), and a behavioral health screen.

experienced possibly concussive events, such as falls or injury from an improvised explosion device. In 2008, the Army began requiring the use of MACE "as soon as tactically possible" for service members exposed to a potential TBI-causing event (Agimi et al., 2018). The 2008 NDAA (Pub. L. 110-181, National Defense Authorization Act for Fiscal Year 2008, January 28, 2008) permitted differential diagnoses of TBI and authorized a pilot to improve its detection, including a computer-based neurocognitive assessment called Automated Neurocognitive Assessment Metrics. Then, in 2010, DTM 09-033, "Policy Guidance for Management of Concussion/Mild Traumatic Brain Injury in the Deployed Setting," was issued for all Services and specified that in deployed settings, commanding officers are required to use MACE to screen service members who are exposed to potentially concussive events. DTM 09-033 also requires the use of the Blast Exposure and Concussion Incident Reporting System for reporting.

Directive-Type Memorandum (DTM) 09-033 was canceled in 2012 but was incorporated into DODI 6490.11, "DoD Policy Guidance for Management of Mild Traumatic Brain Injury/Concussion in the Deployed Setting," on September 18, 2012.

Changes to Disability Evaluation of Posttraumatic Stress Disorder

As noted throughout this report, multiple forces led to changes in both the identification and treatment of PTSD and TBI and to DES. During this time, there was also specific attention on the intersection of these changes—how service members with PTSD and TBI were evaluated for disability and medical retirement. In this section we detail some of the events that led to changes to assessment of PTSD and to assigning a disability rating and determining compensation. As described previously (in Chapter 2), DoDI 1332.39 (1996), *Application of the Veterans Administration Schedule for Rating Disabilities*, specified that service members determined to be unfit because of "mental health disorders due to traumatic stress" (e.g., PTSD) were to receive a minimum 50 percent disability rating and be placed on TDRL. In 2008, a class action lawsuit, *Sabo v. United States*, was brought by OEF and OIF veterans who had been separated, in whole or in part, for unfitness due to PTSD (102 Fed. Cl. 619, 2011). The lawsuit alleged the departments had "failed to assign plaintiffs disability ratings of at least 50 percent when the appropriate Physical Evaluation Board found them unfit for duty due, at least in part, to PTSD." The court accepted the proposed settlement agreement, the key terms of which were that

> a class member who was not placed on the TDRL after separation or retirement will have his or her military records changed to reflect that he or she was placed on the TDRL and was given a 50 [percent] disability rating for PTSD for the first six months following his or her separation or retirement. . . . A class member who was placed on the TDRL will have his or her military records changed to reflect that he or she received a 50 [percent] disability rating for PTSD for the entire time he or she was on the TDRL (Sabo v. United States, 2011).

More than 4,300 veterans of OEF and OIF who had been diagnosed with PTSD were invited to join the class action and benefit from the negotiated settlement, which promised an upgrade in the veteran's disability rating and an expedited review by a military correction board to determine the full extent of the rating improvement (Farray, 2010). PDBR conducted these reviews.

In addition to the *Sabo v. United States* legal case, investigation into problems at individual installations also played a role in changing the way that those with PTSD were managed during disability evaluation. In 2011, media reports found that between 2007 and 2011, more than 40 percent of service members who were being evaluated in DES for PTSD had their diagnoses reconsidered or changed (Moisse, 2012). In response, Congress introduced legislation to require a review of these cases (H.R. 975, 2013). Although the legislation was not passed into law, approximately 431 soldiers had their cases reviewed by PDBR, and the diagnosis was changed for 267 soldiers, approximately 158 of whom had PTSD (Ashton, 2013a, 2013b). While the review of cases was open to all service branches, the Army submitted the vast majority; the Navy submitted only nine cases for review.[5]

---

[5]   Physical Disability Board of Review, personal communication with authors, December 2017.

In response to the investigation and subsequent case review, Army Medical Command Chief of Staff Herbert Coley released a memo that included new guidelines for diagnosing PTSD (DA, 2012). Because the Army and VA observed that service members often do not admit feeling fear or a sense of helplessness, either because of stigma or because of training to overcome these feelings, the guidelines de-emphasized the criteria of feeling "fear, helplessness or horror" (Ashton, 2013a). In addition, the Secretary of the Army issued a directive in May 2012 to "take a holistic look and identify systemic breakdowns or concerns in the [IDES] as they affect the diagnosis and evaluation of [behavioral health] conditions" (U.S. Army, 2013, p. 7). This led to the creation of the Army Task Force on Behavioral Health (ATFBH), which published its corrective action plan (CAP) in January 2013. Prior to the publication of CAP, but during the investigation, ATFBH recommended that the Army proactively implement several initiatives. These resulted in the Army Physical Disability Agency (responsible for administering the PEB phase of DES) increasing its capacity by 2.5 times over six months to 4,000 cases per month, the Army Medical Command improving its Narrative Summary (a stage of MEB during which a written summary of the service member's medical condition[s] is constructed) capacity from an average of 60 days to 30.8 days, and more soldiers completing the IDES process than prior to the implementation of these initiatives (U.S. Army, 2013).

Following the publication of the ATFBH recommendations, the Pentagon published additional guidelines that borrowed language from the Army document and recommended a standardized approach to defining PTSD across all service branches. According to the guidelines, the standardized approach to PTSD must include therapy, even if medication is given. Evaluation should not be overly concerned with malingering or embellishment of symptoms, and the guidelines reiterated de-emphasizing feelings of "fear, hopelessness or horror" as diagnostic criteria (Ashton, 2013a).

There were also incidents at Fort Carson that catalyzed changes to the disability system. As early as 2009 media reports claimed that soldiers at Fort Carson were being "chaptered out," meaning they were being discharged for disorderly conduct with a less than honorable discharge despite the fact that they were complaining of mental health symptoms and had been exposed to traumatic situations. In media coverage, soldiers explained they believed this was happening because for DoD, it was faster and easier to issue a less than honorable discharge (Zwerdling, 2015). The Navy and Air Force have not been immune to these criticisms. For example, a class action lawsuit against the Navy was introduced in 2018 by Marine Corps veterans who felt they had received dishonorable discharges when their problems were due to PTSD (Philipps, 2018).

In 2016, DoD conducted an internal review of its policies and processes regarding administrative separations and finding some inconsistencies across the service branches (DoD, 2016). Following that review, in 2017, GAO issued a report stating that 16 percent of service members who were separated for misconduct had been diagnosed with PTSD or TBI. When other conditions that could possibly result from deployment were added to the analysis, it included 62 percent of those who were separated for misconduct (GAO, 2017, p. 12). The report highlighted issues with Air Force and Navy policies related to screening for PTSD and TBI prior to separation for misconduct. To address these issues, the Secretary of the Air Force launched the Invisible Wounds Initiative in 2016, focused on improving care for airmen with PTSD and/or TBI. In addition to efforts aimed at improving education and training, culture, process, policy, and care delivery, the program established an Interim Medical Review Panel to ensure individuals going through IDES received evidence-based care for these conditions (Pflanz, 2017).

In August 2017, DoD issued new guidance for how review boards were to consider cases involving PTSD, TBI, and other mental health conditions (DoD OUSD[P&R], 2017). In addition, DoD and VA developed an online tool to make it easier for veterans with "bad paper" discharges to request a review of their discharge status (DoD, 2018).

A timeline of major events between 1997 and 2018 that impacted the management of mental health issues among service members is presented below in Figure 3.1.

Figure 3.1
Timeline of Major Mental Health Policies and Legal Actions, 1997–2018

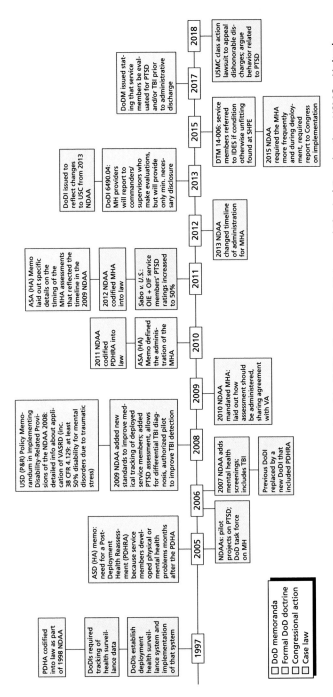

NOTES: OIE = Operation Iraqi Freedom; MH = mental health; SHPE = Separation History and Physical Examination; USMC = United States Marine Corps.

CHAPTER FOUR

Summary and Conclusion

The primary goal of this report was to describe the major policy changes relevant to DES as well as the diagnosis, treatment, and disability evaluation of PTSD and TBI from 2001 to 2018. To do this, we conducted a review of the relevant laws, regulations, and policy doctrine; identified the motivations and impetus for policy changes through a review of reports, journal articles, briefings, news articles, and other sources; and met with stakeholders involved in either policy-making or the implementation of IDES.

DES, created in 1947, was set forth in lengthy and explicit doctrine in 1996 (10 U.S.C. §1201, 2008; DoDI 1332.39, 1996), only a few years before the onset of the wars in Iraq and Afghanistan, and the system quickly faced unexpected challenges in terms of both the number of service members being processed and the unique mental and behavioral health concerns they faced, notably PTSD and TBI. Since 2001, there have been several changes to the way service members are evaluated for disability, most notably the transition from LDES to IDES in 2011, following several years of a pilot program. The goal of IDES was to streamline the disability evaluation process and reduce confusion among service members facing medical discharge. The primary innovation was the introduction of a "single set of disability medical examinations appropriate for fitness determination by the Military Departments and a single set of disability ratings provided by VA for appropriate use by both departments" (DoD OUSD[P&R], 2011, p. 10). IDES also reduced variation in DES policies across services, such as requiring all services to meet the same timeliness standard.[1] In implementing IDES, DoD policy specified that service members diagnosed with a mental disorder due to traumatic stress would be placed on TDRL with a 50 percent disability rating and reevaluated periodically. Legal challenges, including a class action lawsuit, brought attention to this policy and the need for consistent application.

Further refinements and changes have been made to the disability system since the introduction of IDES. First, there has been a movement back toward the legacy system, where service members injured in initial training or on-duty-related cases may be evaluated under LDES; this is also the case where processing through IDES could be detrimental. The option to be evaluated under the legacy system was intended to allow service members who were injured during initial training to be processed out of the military quickly rather than spending nearly a year in IDES. Second, the policy on administrative separations was updated in 2014, adding an additional requirement for separation health assessments to ensure that service members with PTSD or TBI were appropriately screened and treated before separation. In 2017, the guidance on TDRL was updated, reducing the maximum length of time a member remains on the list from five years to three years. This was in response to research that found the overwhelming majority of service members who were on TDRL for more than three years were permanently retired (DoD OUSD[P&R], undated). And in recent years, there has been attention to improving the timeliness of the DES process in response a GAO report on the issue (GAO, 2012).

During this same period, policies have been created and revised around the identification and treatment of PTSD and TBI, the two signature injuries of the wars in Iraq and Afghanistan. In terms of screening, the PDHRA was introduced in 2006, in recognition of the potential for delayed onset of physical and mental health problems in returning service members. Enhanced mental health and TBI screen-

---

[1] Despite standardization in policy through IDES, there necessarily remain differences across services in DES processes; for example, the Army MEB determines whether soldiers meet Army medical retention standards, while the Navy does not have medical retention standards and uses other criteria to determine fitness for duty.

ing tools were added to both the PDHA and PDHRA. In addition, the MHA, an assessment specifically directed at the identification of mental health conditions, was introduced in 2011 and then updated in 2013 and 2014.

Evaluation for disability in the military is a complex process, involving the decision to refer a service member for evaluation, assessment of his or her medical condition, and decisions about retention standards and fitness for duty, disability ratings, and in the case of temporary retirement, subsequent evaluations until the condition or conditions stabilize. Furthermore, successful management of invisible wounds such as PTSD and TBI requires early and frequent screening, accurate diagnoses, and effective treatment options, while maintaining a holistic view of the service member's needs, behaviors, and outcomes.

As this report has described, there have been major changes not only to DES itself but also, simultaneously, to the understanding and treatment of PTSD and TBI during the time period 2001–2018. The companion report to this one describes trends in diagnoses of PTSD and TBI over this time period, along with trends in disability evaluation outcomes, such as disability ratings and final dispositions (Krull et al., 2021). This report provides context for those trends, although it is not possible to assign causality. As this report makes clear, changes to how disability evaluation was conducted and how service members with PTSD or TBI were identified and treated occurred together, resulting in a new landscape for assessing and evaluating these signature injuries of the Iraq and Afghanistan wars.

References

Acosta, Joie D., Amariah Becker, Jennifer L. Cerully, Michael P. Fisher, Laurie T. Martin, Raffaele Vardavas, Mary Ellen Slaughter, and Terry L. Schell, *Mental Health Stigma in the Military*, Santa Monica, Calif.: RAND Corporation, RR-426-OSD, 2014a.

Acosta, Joie D., Kerry Reynolds, Emily M. Gillen, Kevin Carter Feeney, Carrie M. Farmer, and Robin M. Weinick, *The RAND Online Measure Repository for Evaluating Psychological Health and Traumatic Brain Injury Programs: The RAND Toolkit, Volume 2*, Santa Monica, Calif.: RAND Corporation, RR-487/2-OSD, 2014b. As of May 16, 2019: https://www.rand.org/pubs/research_reports/RR487z2.html

Acosta, Joie D., Wenjing Huang, Maria Orlando Edelen, Jennifer L. Cerully, Sarah Soliman, and Anita Chandra, *Measuring Barriers to Mental Health Care in the Military: The RAND Barriers and Facilitators to Care Item Banks*, Santa Monica, Calif.: RAND Corporation, RR-1762-OSD, 2018. As of May 15, 2019: https://www.rand.org/pubs/research_reports/RR1762.html

Agimi, Yll, Lemma Ebssa Regasa, Brian Ivins, Saafan Malik, Katherine Helmick, and Donald Marion, "Role of Department of Defense Policies in Identifying Traumatic Brain Injuries Among Deployed US Service Members, 2001–2016," *American Journal of Public Health*, Vol. 108, No. 5, 2018, pp. 683–688.

Ashton, Adam, "Pentagon Reworks PTSD Strategy," *McClatchy DC Bureau*, February 19, 2013a. As of May 16, 2019: http://www.mcclatchydc.com/news/nation-world/national/article24745132.html

Ashton, Adam, "Investigation: Culture of Shortchanging Soldiers on PTSD Didn't Exist at Madigan Hospital," *McClatchy DC Bureau*, March 18, 2013b. As of May 16, 2019: http://www.mcclatchydc.com/news/nation-world/world/article24746824.html

ASD(HA)—*See* Assistant Secretary of Defense for Health Affairs.

Assistant Secretary of Defense for Health Affairs, "Post-Deployment Health Reassessment," memorandum, Washington, D.C., March 10, 2005a.

———, "Mental Health Assessments for Members of the Armed Forces Deployed in Connection with a Contingency Operation," memorandum, Washington, D.C., July 19, 2010.

———, "Directive-Type Memorandum 11-011: Mental Health Assessments for Members of the Military Services Deployed in Connection with a Contingency Operation," Washington, D.C., August 12, 2011.

———, "Post-Deployment Health Reassessment," memorandum, Washington, D.C., March 10, 2005b.

Baker, Peter, "At Walter Reed, Bush Offers an Apology," *Washington Post*, March 30, 2007.

Benjamin, Mark, "Sick, Wounded Troops Held in Squalor," United Press International, October 17, 2003.

Blakeley, Katherine, and Don J. Jansen, *Post-Traumatic Stress Disorder and Other Mental Health Problems in the Military: Oversight Issues for Congress*, Washington, D.C.: Congressional Research Service, August 8, 2013.

Bliese, Paul D., Kathleen M. Wright, Jeffrey L. Thomas, Amy B. Adler, and Charles W. Hoge, *Screening for Traumatic Stress Among Re-Deploying Soldiers (U.S. Army Medical Research Unit-Europe Research Report 2004-001)*, Heidelberg, Germany: USAMRU-E, 2004.

Boivin, Michael R., Paul O. Kwon, David N. Cowan, Elizabeth R. Packnett, Amanda L. Piccirillo, and Hoda Elmasry, *Disability Evaluation Systems Analysis and Research: Annual Report 2015*, Silver Spring, Md., 2015. As of May 15, 2019: https://apps.dtic.mil/dtic/tr/fulltext/u2/1005611.pdf

Carey, Benedict, "The Struggle to Gauge a War's Psychological Cost," *New York Times*, November 26, 2005. As of May 15, 2019: https://www.nytimes.com/2005/11/26/health/the-struggle-to-gauge-a-wars -psychological-cost.html

CDC—*See* Centers for Disease Control and Prevention.

Centers for Disease Control and Prevention, "Traumatic Brain Injury and Concussion," web page, March 4, 2019. As of July 19, 2019: https://www.cdc.gov/traumaticbraininjury/index.html

CFR—*See* Code of Federal Regulations.

Christensen, Eric, Joyce McMahon, Elizabeth Schaefer, Ted Jaditz, and Dan Harris, *Final Report for the Veterans' Disability Benefits Commission: Compensation, Survey Results, and Selected Topics*, Alexandria, Va.: The CNA Corporation, August 2007.

Code of Federal Regulations, Title 38, Section 4.129, Mental Disorders Due to Traumatic Stress, 1996a.

Code of Federal Regulations, Title 38, Sections 4.40–4.130, Disability Ratings, 1996b.

Curtain, Neil P., *DOD Needs to Improve Force Health Protection and Surveillance Processes*, Testimony Before the Committee on Veterans' Affairs, House of Representatives, Washington, D.C.: General Accounting Office, GAO-04-158T, October 16, 2003.

DA—*See* U.S. Department of the Army.

Defense Manpower Data Center, *CTS Deployment File Baseline Report*, Seaside, Calif., February 28, 2018.

Department of Defense Directive Type Memorandum 09-033, "Policy Guidance for Management of Concussion/ Mild Traumatic Brain Injury in the Deployed Setting," June 21, 2010

Department of Defense Instruction 1332.14, *Enlisted Administrative Separations*, Washington, D.C.: U.S. Department of Defense, January 27, 2014.

Department of Defense Instruction 1332.18, *Disability Evaluation System*, Washington, D.C.: U.S. Department of Defense, August 5, 2014.

Department of Defense Instruction 1332.18, *Disability Evaluation System*, Washington, D.C.: U.S. Department of Defense, incorporating change 1, May 17, 2018.

Department of Defense Instruction 1332.18, *Disability Evaluation System*, Appendix 4 to Enclosure 3, Washington, D.C.: U.S. Department of Defense, May 17, 2018.

Department of Defense Instruction 1332.38, *Physical Disability Evaluation*, Washington, D.C.: U.S. Department of Defense, November 14, 1996.

Department of Defense Instruction 1332.39, *Application of the Veterans Administration Schedule for Rating Disabilities*, Washington, D.C.: U.S. Department of Defense, November 14, 1996.

Department of Defense Instruction 6040.44, *Lead DoD Component for the Physical Disability Board of Review (PDBR)*, Washington, D.C.: U.S. Department of Defense, June 27, 2008.

Department of Defense Instruction 6040.44, *Lead DoD Component for the Physical Disability Board of Review (PDBR)*, Washington, D.C.: U.S. Department of Defense, June 2, 2015.

Department of Defense Instruction 6200.06, *Periodic Health Assessment (PHA) Program*, Washington, D.C.: U.S. Department of Defense, September 8, 2016.

Department of Defense Instruction 6490.2, *Joint Medical Surveillance*, Washington, D.C.: U.S. Department of Defense, August 30, 1997.

Department of Defense Instruction 6490.3, *Implementation and Application of Joint Medical Surveillance for Deployments*, Washington, D.C.: U.S. Department of Defense, August 7, 1997.

Department of Defense Instruction 6490.03, *Deployment Health*, Washington, D.C.: U.S. Department of Defense, August 11, 2006.

Department of Defense Instruction 6490.11, *DoD Policy Guidance for Management of Mild Traumatic Brain Injury/Concussion in the Deployed Setting*, Washington, D.C.: U.S. Department of Defense, September 18, 2012.

Department of Defense Instruction 6490.12, *Mental Health Assessments for Service Members Deployed in Connection with a Contingency Operation*, Washington, D.C.: U.S. Department of Defense, February 26, 2013.

Department of Defense Manual 1332.18, *Disability Evaluation System (DES) Manual: General Information and Legacy Disability Evaluation System (LDES) Time Standards*, vol. 1, Washington, D.C.: U.S. Department of Defense, August 5, 2014a.

Department of Defense Manual 1332.18, *Disability Evaluation System (DES) Manual: Integrated Disability Evaluation System (IDES)*, vol. 2, Washington, D.C.: U.S. Department of Defense, August 5, 2014b.

Department of Defense, Office of the General Counsel, Memorandum on Effect of Section 1642 of the National Defense Authorization Act for Fiscal Year 2008 on DoDI 1332.29, March 17, 2008.

DoD—*See* U.S. Department of Defense.

DoDM—*See* Department of Defense Manual.

DoD OUSD(P&R)—*See* U.S. Department of Defense, Office of the Under Secretary of Defense (Personnel and Readiness).

Emery, Erin, "Ft. Carson on Defensive After Soldiers Report PTSD Stigma," *Denver Post*, December 25, 2006. As of May 16, 2019:
https://www.denverpost.com/2006/12/25/ft-carson-on-defensive-after-soldiers-report-ptsd-stigma/

Farmer, Carrie M., Heather Krull, Thomas W. Concannon, Molly Simmons, Francesca Pillemer, Teague Ruder, Andrew M. Parker, Maulik P. Purohit, Liisa Hiatt, Benjamin Batorsky, and Kimberly A. Hepner, *Understanding Treatment of Mild Traumatic Brain Injury in the Military Health System*, Santa Monica, Calif.: RAND Corporation, RR-844-OSD, 2016. As of July 19, 2019:
https://www.rand.org/pubs/research_reports/RR844.html

Farray, Yanira, "Class Action Suit to Yield Benefits for Thousands of Veterans," *Veterans Today*, February 20, 2010. As of May 16, 2019:
https://www.veteranstodayarchives.com/2010/02/20/class-action-suit-to-yield-benefits-to-1000s-of-veterans/

GAO—*See* U.S. Government Accountability Office.

Headquarters, Department of the Army, *EXORD 080-12: Army Disability Evaluation System (DES) Standardization*, Washington, D.C., February 2012.

Hepner, Kimberly A., Coreen Farris, Carrie M. Farmer, Praise O. Iyiewuare, Terri Tanielian, Asa Wilks, Michael Robbins, Susan M. Paddock, and Harold Alan Pincus, *Delivering Clinical Practice Guideline–Concordant Care for PTSD and Major Depression in Military Treatment Facilities*, Santa Monica, Calif.: RAND Corporation, RR-1692-OSD, 2017a. As of May 16, 2019:
https://www.rand.org/pubs/research_reports/RR1692.html

Hepner, Kimberly A., Carol P. Roth, Elizabeth M. Sloss, Susan M. Paddock, Praise O. Iyiewuare, Martha J. Timmer, and Harold Alan Pincus, *Quality of Care for PTSD and Depression in the Military Health System: Final Report*, Santa Monica, Calif.: RAND Corporation, RR-1542-OSD, 2017b. As of May 16, 2019:
https://www.rand.org/pubs/research_reports/RR1542.html

Hoge, Charles W., Jennifer L. Auchterlonie, and Charles S. Milliken, "Mental Health Problems, Use of Mental Health Services, and Attrition from Military Service After Returning from Deployment to Iraq or Afghanistan," *Journal of the American Medical Association*, Vol. 295, No. 9, 2006, pp. 1023–1032.

Hoge, Charles W., Carl A. Castro, Stephen C. Messer, Dennis McGurk, Dave I. Cotting, and Robert L. Koffman, "Combat Duty in Iraq and Afghanistan, Mental Health Problems, and Barriers to Care," *New England Journal of Medicine,* Vol. 351, No. 1, 2004, pp. 13–22.

Hoge, Charles W., Herb M. Goldberg, and Carl A. Castro, "Care of War Veterans with Mild Traumatic Brain Injury—Flawed Perspectives," *New England Journal of Medicine*, Vol. 360, No. 16, 2009, pp. 1588–1591.

Hoge, Charles W., Dennis McGurk, Jeffrey L. Thomas, Anthony L. Cox, Charles C. Engel, and Carl A. Castro, "Mild Traumatic Brain Injury in U.S. Soldiers Returning from Iraq," *New England Journal of Medicine*, Vol. 358, No. 5, 2008, pp. 453-463.

H.R. 975, Servicemember Mental Health Review Act, March 5, 2013.

H.R. 1685, Honor Our Commitment Act, March 22, 2017.

Hull, Anne, "Wounded or Disabled but Still on Active Duty," *Washington Post*, December 1, 2004, p. A23.

Independent Review Group, *Rehabilitative Care and Administrative Processes at Walter Reed Army Medical Center and National Naval Medical Center*, Arlington, Va., April 2007.

Institute of Medicine, *Posttraumatic Stress Disorder: Diagnosis and Assessment*, Washington, D.C.: National Academies Press, 2006. As of May 15, 2019:
https://www.nap.edu/catalog/11674/posttraumatic-stress-disorder-diagnosis-and -assessment

————, *PTSD Compensation and Military Service*, Washington, D.C.: National Academies Press, May 8, 2007a. As of May 15, 2019:
https://www.nap.edu/catalog/11870/ptsd-compensation-and-military-service

————, *Treatment of PTSD: An Assessment of the Evidence*, Washington, D.C.: National Academies Press, October 17, 2007b. As of May 15, 2019:
https://www.nap.edu/catalog/11955/treatment-of-posttraumatic-stress-disorder -an-assessment-of-the-evidence

————, *Treatment for Posttraumatic Stress Disorder in Military and Veteran Populations: Final Assessment*, Washington, D.C.: June 20, 2014.

IOM—*See* Institute of Medicine.

Krull, Heather, Carrie Farmer, Stephanie Rennane, Evan Goldstein, Philip Armour, and Teague Ruder, *Trends in Department of Defense Disability Evaluation System Ratings and Awards for Posttraumatic Stress Disorder (PTSD) and Traumatic Brain Injury, 2001–2017*, Santa Monica, Calif.: RAND Corporation, RR-3174-OSD, 2021.

Mann, Christopher T., *U.S. War Costs, Casualties, and Personnel Levels Since 9/11*, Washington, D.C.: Congressional Research Service, IF11182, April 18, 2019. As of July 19, 2019:
https://fas.org/sgp/crs/natsec/IF11182.pdf

Marcum, Cheryl Y., Robert M. Emmerichs, Jennifer Sloane McCombs, and Harry J. Thie, *Methods and Actions for Improving Performance of the Department of Defense Disability Evaluation System*, Santa Monica, Calif.: RAND Corporation, MR-1228, 2002. As of May 16, 2019:
https://www.rand.org/pubs/monograph_reports/MR1228.html

Martin, Laurie T., Coreen Farris, David M. Adamson, and Robin M. Weinick, *A Systematic Process to Facilitate Evidence-Informed Decisionmaking Regarding Program Expansion: The RAND Toolkit, Volume 3*, Santa Monica, Calif.: RAND Corporation, RR-487/3-OSD, 2014. As of May 16, 2019:
https://www.rand.org/pubs/research_reports/RR487z3.html

McGeary, Michael, Morgan A. Ford, Susan R. McCutchen, and David K. Barnes, eds., *A 21st Century System for Evaluating Veterans for Disability Benefits*, Washington, D.C.: National Academies Press, 2007, pp. 69–81.

Military Health System, "Integrated Disability Evaluation System," web page, undated(a). As of May 15, 2019:
https://www.health.mil/Military-Health-Topics/Conditions-and-Treatments/ Physical-Disability/Disability-Evaluation/Integrated-Evaluation-System

————, "Periodic Health Assessment," web page, undated(b). As of July 19, 2019:
https://health.mil/Military-Health-Topics/Health-Readiness/Reserve-Health -Readiness-Program/Our-Services/PHA

Milliken, Charles S., Jennifer L. Auchterlonie, and Charles W. Hoge, "Longitudinal Assessment of Mental Health Problems Among Active and Reserve Component Soldiers Returning from the Iraq War," *Journal of the American Medical Association*, Vol. 298, No. 18, 2007, pp. 2141–2148.

Moisse, Katie, "Army Hospital Accused of Reversing PTSD Diagnoses to Cut Costs," *ABC News*, March 22, 2012. As of May 16, 2019:
http://abcnews.go.com/Health/MindMoodNews/madigan-army-medical-center
-investigation-reneging-ptsd-care/story?id=15969914

National Veterans Legal Services Program, "Sabo v. United States: OIF and OEF Veterans with Post Traumatic Stress Disorder (PTSD)," web page, 2019. As of May 16, 2019:
http://www.nvlsp.org/what-we-do/class-actions/sabo-ptsd-lawsuit.

Obama, Barack, "Executive Order: Improving Access to Mental Health Services for Veterans, Service Members, and Military Families," Washington, D.C.: The White House, Office of the Press Secretary, August 31, 2012.

Office of the Secretary of Defense, Mental Health Assessments for Members of the Armed Forces, Required by: Section 701 of the Carl Levin and Howard P. "Buck" McKeon National Defense Authorization Act for Fiscal Year 2015 (Public Law 113-291), Washington, D.C.: U.S. Department of Defense, January 11, 2018.

OIF MHAT—See *Operation Iraqi Freedom (OIF) Mental Health Advisory Team (MHAT) Report.*

Operation Iraqi Freedom (OIF) Mental Health Advisory Team (MHAT) Report, December 16, 2003. As of May 15, 2019:
https://www.globalsecurity.org/military/library/report/2004/mhat_report.pdf

Pflanz, Steven, "Presentation to the Subcommittee on Military Personnel Committee on Armed Services United States House of Representatives," Washington, D.C.: Department of the Air Force, United States Air Force Medical Support Agency, April 27, 2017.

Philipps, Dave, "Suit Calls Navy Board Biased Against Veterans with PTSD," *New York Times*, March 2, 2018. As of May 16, 2019:
https://www.nytimes.com/2018/03/02/us/navy-ptsd-lawsuit.html

The President's Commission on Care for America's Returning Wounded Warriors, *Serve, Support, Simplify*, Washington, D.C., July 2007. As of July 19, 2019:
http://www.patriotoutreach.org/docs/presidents-commission-report-july-2007.pdf

The President's Task Force to Improve Health Care Delivery for Our Nation's Veterans, *Final Report*, Washington, D.C., May 2003.

Priest, Dana, and Anne Hull, "Soldiers Face Neglect, Frustration at Army's Top Medical Facility," *Washington Post*, February 18, 2007.

Prins, Annabel, Paige Ouimette, Rachel Kimerling, Rebecca P., Cameron, Daniela S. Hugelshofer, Jennifer Shaw-Hegwer, Ann Thraikill, Fred D. Gusman, and Javald I. Sheikh, "The Primary Care PTSD Screen (PC-PTSD): Development and Operating Characteristics," *Primary Care Psychiatry*, Vol. 9, No. 1, 2003, pp. 9–14.

Public Law 105-85, National Defense Authorization Act for Fiscal Year 1998, November 18, 1997.

Public Law 107-314, National Defense Authorization Act for Fiscal Year 2003, December 2, 2002.

Public Law 108-136, National Defense Authorization Act for Fiscal Year 2004, November 24, 2003.

Public Law 109-364, National Defense Authorization Act for Fiscal Year 2007, October 17, 2006.

Public Law 110-181, National Defense Authorization Act for Fiscal Year 2008, January 28, 2008.

Public Law 111-84, National Defense Authorization Act for Fiscal Year 2010, October 28, 2009.

Public Law 112-81, National Defense Authorization Act for Fiscal Year 2012, December 31, 2011.

Public Law 111-383, Division A, Title VII, Ike Skelton National Defense Authorization Act for Fiscal Year 2011, January 7, 2011.

Public Law 112-239, National Defense Authorization Act for Fiscal Year 2013, January 2, 2013.

Public Law 113-291, Carl Levin and Howard P. "Buck" McKeon National Defense Authorization Act for Fiscal Year 2015, December 19, 2014.

Public Law 114-328, National Defense Authorization Act for Fiscal Year 2017, Subpart C, Section 525, Reduction of Tenure on the Temporary Disability Retired List, November 30, 2016.

Rostker, Bernard, *Providing for the Casualties of War: The American Experience Through World War II*, Santa Monica, Calif.: RAND Corporation, MG-1164-OSD, 2013. As of April 23, 2019:
https://www.rand.org/pubs/monographs/MG1164.html

Ryan, Gery W., Carrie M. Farmer, David M. Adamson, and Robin M. Weinick, *A Program Manager's Guide for Program Improvement in Ongoing Psychological Health and Traumatic Brain Injury Programs: The RAND Toolkit, Volume 4*, Santa Monica, Calif.: RAND Corporation, RR-487/4-OSD, 2014. As of May 16, 2019:
https://www.rand.org/pubs/research_reports/RR487z4.html

S. 1606, Dignified Treatment of Wounded Warriors Act, Washington, D.C., July 25, 2007.

Sabo v. United States, 102 Federal Claim 619, 2011.

Seal, Karen H., Daneile Bertenthal, Christian R. Miner, Saunak Sen, and Charles Marmar, "Bringing the War Back Home: Mental Health Disorders Among 103,788 U.S. Veterans Returning from Iraq and Afghanistan Seen at Department of Veterans Affairs Facilities," *Archives of Internal Medicine*, Vol. 167, No. 5, 2007, pp. 476–482.

Simmons, Molly MacMhathan, *The Integrated Disability Evaluation System; The Political Life Cycle of Health Policy from Concept to Evaluation*, dissertation, Baltimore, Md.: Johns Hopkins University, 2015.

Tanielian, Terri, and Lisa H. Jaycox, eds., *Invisible Wounds of War: Psychological and Cognitive Injuries, Their Consequences, and Services to Assist Recovery*, Santa Monica, Calif.: RAND Corporation, MG-720-CCF, 2008. As of May 13, 2019: https://www.rand.org/pubs/monographs/MG720.html.

Tanielian, Terri, Lisa H. Jaycox, Terry L. Schell, Grant N. Marshall, M. Audrey Burnam, Christine Eibner, Benjamin Karney, Lisa S. Meredith, Jeanne S. Ringel, and Mary E. Vaiana, *Invisible Wounds of War: Summary and Recommendations for Addressing Psychological and Cognitive Injuries*, Santa Monica, Calif.: RAND Corporation, MG-720/1-CCF, 2008. As of May 13, 2019: https://www.rand.org/pubs/monographs/MG720z1.html

Task Force on Returning Global War on Terror Heroes, *Report to the President*, Washington, D.C., April 19, 2007.

U.S. Army, Army Task Force on Behavioral Health, *Corrective Action Plan*, Washington, D.C., January 2013.

U.S. Army Medical Command, *IDES Guidebook: An Overview of the Integrated Disability Evaluation System*, San Antonio, Tex., July 2013.

U.S. Code, Title 10, Chapter 61, Retirement or Separation for Physical Disability, 2011.

U.S. Code, Title 10, Section 1074f, Medical Tracking System for Members Deployed Overseas, 2012.

U.S. Code, Title 10, Section 1201, Regulars and Members on Active Duty For More Than 30 Days: Retirement, 2008.

U.S. Code, Title 10, Section 1210, Members on Temporary Disability Retired List: Periodic Physical Examination; Final Determination of Status, 2017.

U.S. Code, Title 10, Section 1214a, Members Determined Fit for Duty in Physical Evaluation Board: Prohibition on Involuntary Administrative Separation or Denial of Reenlistment due to Unsuitability Based on Medical Conditions Considered in Evaluation, 2011.

U.S. Code, Title 10, Section 1216a, Determinations of Disability: Requirements and Limitations on Determinations, 2008.

U.S. Code, Title 10, Section 1218, Discharge or Release from Active Duty: Claims for Compensation, Pension, or Hospitalization, 2008.

U.S. Code, Title 10, Section 1554, Review of Retirement or Separation without Pay for Physical Disability, 2011.

U.S. Department of the Army, "Policy Guidance on the Assessment and Treatment of Post-Traumatic Stress Disorder (PTSD)," OTSG/MEDCOM Policy Memorandum 12-035 (subsequently revised as 14-094 and 18-018), Fort Sam Houston, Tex., April 10, 2012.

U.S. Department of Defense, "Defense Centers of Excellence for Psychological Health and Traumatic Brain Injury, Annual Report 2009," Bethesda, Md., 2009. As of July 28, 2019:
https://apps.dtic.mil/dtic/tr/fulltext/u2/a523055.pdf

U.S. Department of Defense, "DoD Directives Division," web page, undated. As of May 15, 2019:
http://www.dtic.mil/whs/directives/index.html

———, Deployment Mental Health Assessment (MHA), DD Form 2900, Washington, D.C.: Executive Services Directorate, June 2005.

———, Post-Deployment Health Assessment (PDHA), DD Form 2795, Washington, D.C.: Executive Services Directorate, September 2012.

———, Post-Deployment Health Assessment (PDHA), DD Form 2796, Washington, D.C.: Executive Services Directorate, October 2015.

———, "DoD Announces New Outreach Efforts to Veterans Regarding Discharges and Military Records," press release, December 30, 2016. As of July 19, 2019:
https://dod.defense.gov/News/News-Releases/News-Release-View/Article/1039945/dod-announces-new-outreach-efforts-to-veterans-regarding-discharges-and-militar/

———, "DoD and VA Release Online Tool to Assist Veterans with Discharge Upgrade Process," press release, January 25, 2018.

———, Defense Casualty Analysis System, "U.S. Military Casualties–Operation Freedom's Sentinel (OFS) Wounded in Action," web page, July 18, 2019. As of July 19, 2019:
https://dcas.dmdc.osd.mil/dcas/pages/report_ofs_wound.xhtml

U.S. Department of Defense, Office of the Under Secretary of Defense (Personnel and Readiness), *Disability Evaluation System (DES) Pilot Operations Manual*, Washington, D.C.: U.S. Department of Defense, November 2008.

U.S. Department of Defense, Office of the Under Secretary of Defense (Personnel and Readiness), "Implementing Disability-Related Provisions of the National Defense Authorization Act of 2008 (Pub 1. 110-181)," memorandum, Washington, D.C., October 14, 2008.

————, "Expedited DES Process for Members with Catastrophic Conditions and Combat-Related Stress," memorandum, Washington, D.C., January 6, 2009.

————, "Clarifying Guidance to Military Discharge Review Boards and Boards for Correction of Military/Naval Records Considering Requests by Veterans for Modifications of Their Discharge Due to Mental Health Conditions, Sexual Assault, or Sexual Harassment," memorandum, Washington, D.C., August 25, 2017.

U.S. Department of Defense, Task Force on Mental Health, *The Department of Defense Plan to Achieve the Vision of the DoD Task Force on Mental Health*, Washington, D.C., September 19, 2007. As of May 15, 2019: https://www.pdhealth.mil/department-defense-plan-achieve-vision-dod-task -force-mental-health

U.S. Department of Defense, Office of the Under Secretary of Defense (Personnel and Readiness), "The Temporary Disability Retired List (TDRL): An Assessment of Its Continuing Utility and Future Role," Washington, D.C., undated.

————, "Policy and Procedural Update for the Disability Evaluation System (DES) Pilot Program," Washington, D.C., December 11, 2008.

————, "Directive-Type Memorandum (DTM) 10-022—Implementing Required Medical Exam Before Administrative Separation for Post-Traumatic Stress Disorder (PTSD) or Traumatic Brain Injury (TBI)," Washington, D.C., July 25, 2010.

————, "Directive-Type Memorandum (DTM) 11-015—Integrated Disability Evaluation System (IDES)," Washington, D.C., December 19, 2011.

————, "Memorandum: Enrollment in the Legacy Disability Evaluation System," Washington, D.C., October 15, 2015.

————, "Revised Timeliness Goals for the Integrated Disability Evaluation System (IDES)," Directive-Type Memorandum DTM-18-004, Washington, D.C., July 30, 2018.

U.S. Department of Defense Warrior Care, "Integrated Disability Evaluation System (IDES)," web page, undated. As of July 19, 2019: https://warriorcare.dodlive.mil/disability-evaluation/integrateddes/

U.S. Department of Veterans Affairs, "Task Force Aims at Improved Services for GWOT Veterans," press release, Washington, D.C.: Office of Public and Intergovernmental Affairs, April 24, 2007. As of July 19, 2019: https://www.va.gov/opa/pressrel/pressrelease.cfm?id=1327

————, National Center for PTSD, "PTSD Consultation Program," web page, 2019a. As of July 19, 2019: https://www.ptsd.va.gov/professional/consult/index.asp

————, "VHA Publications," web page, May 14, 2019b. As of May 15, 2019: https://www.va.gov/vhapublications/

U.S. Department of Veterans Affairs and Department of Defense, "Expansion of the DoD/VA Integrated Pilot Disability Evaluation System (IPDES)—Providing a Single Disability Evaluation/Transition Medical Examination and Single Source Disability Rating," Memorandum of Agreement, Washington, D.C., June 16, 2009.

U.S. Department of Veterans Affairs and Department of Defense Joint Executive Council, *FY 2008 Annual Report*, Washington, D.C., February 2009.

U.S. Government Accountability Office, *VA and Defense Health Care: More Information Needed to Determine If VA Can Meet an Increase in Demand for Post-Traumatic Stress Disorder Services*, Washington, D.C., GAO-04-1069, September 2004a.

———, *Defense Health Care: Force Health Protection and Surveillance Policy Compliance Was Mixed, but Appears Better for Recent Deployments*, Washington, D.C., GAO-05-120, November 12, 2004b.

———, *Military Disability System: Improved Oversight Needed to Ensure Consistent and Timely Outcomes for Reserve and Active Duty Service Members*, Washington, D.C., GAO-06-362, 2006.

———, *Mental Health and Traumatic Brain Injury Screening Efforts Implemented, but Consistent Pre-Deployment Medical Record Review Policies Needed*, Washington, D.C., GAO-08-615, May 30, 2008a.

———, *Defense Health Care: Oversight of Military Services' Post-Deployment Health Reassessment Completion Rates Is Limited*, Washington, D.C., GAO-08-1025R, September 2008b.

———, *Military Disability Retirement: Closer Monitoring Would Improve the Temporary Retirement Process*, Washington, D.C., GAO-09-289, April 13, 2009a.

———, *Post-Deployment Health Reassessment Documentation Needs Improvement*, Washington, D.C., GAO-10-56, November 2009b.

———, *Preliminary Observations on Evaluation and Planned Expansion of DOD/VA Pilot*, Washington, D.C., GAO 11-191T, November 2010a.

———, *Military and Veterans Disability System: Pilot Has Achieved Some Goals, but Further Planning and Monitoring Needed*, Washington, D.C., GAO 11-69, December 2010b.

———, *Military Disability System: Improved Monitoring Needed to Better Track and Manage Performance*, Washington, D.C., GAO-12-676, 2012.

———, *Actions Needed to Ensure Post-Traumatic Stress Disorder and Traumatic Brain Injury Are Considered in Misconduct Separations*, Washington, D.C., GAO 17-260, May 2017.

VA—*See* U.S. Department of Veterans Affairs.

VDBC—*See* Veterans' Disability Benefits Commission.

Veterans' Disability Benefits Commission, *Honoring the Call to Duty: Veterans' Disability Benefits in the 21st Century*, Washington, D.C., October 2007.

Warner, Christopher H., George N. Appenzeller, Thomas Grieger, Slava Belenkiy, Jill Breitbach, Jessica Parker, Carolynn M. Warner, and Charles Hoge, "Importance of Anonymity to Encourage Honest Reporting in Mental Health Screening After Combat Deployment," *Archives of General Psychiatry*, Vol. 68, No. 10, 2011, pp. 1065–1071.

Weathers, Frank W., Brett T. Litz, Terence M. Keane, Patrick A. Palmieri, Brian P. Marx, and Paula P. Schnurr, "The PTSD Checklist for *DSM-5* (PCL-5), 2013," Washington, D.C.: U.S. Department of Veterans Affairs. As of July 19, 2019: https://www.ptsd.va.gov/professional/assessment/adult-sr/ptsd-checklist.asp

Weinick, Robin M., Ellen Burke Beckjord, Carrie M. Farmer, Laurie T. Martin, Emily M. Gillen, Joie D. Acosta, Michael P. Fisher, Jeffrey Garnett, Gabriella C. Gonzalez, Todd C. Helmus, Lisa H. Jaycox, Kerry Reynolds, Nicholas Salcedo, and Deborah M. Scharf, *Programs Addressing Psychological Health and Traumatic Brain Injury Among U.S. Military Servicemembers and Their Families*, Santa Monica, Calif.: RAND Corporation, TR-950-OSD, 2011. As of May 16, 2019: https://www.rand.org/pubs/technical_reports/TR950.html

Welch, William M., "Trauma of Iraq War Haunting Thousands Returning Home," *USA Today*, February 28, 2005.

Zwerdling, Daniel, "Missed Treatment: Soldiers with Mental Health Issues Dismissed for 'Misconduct,'" *All Things Considered*, National Public Radio, October 28, 2015. As of May 16, 2019: https://www.npr.org/2015/10/28/451146230/missed-treatment-soldiers-with -mental-health-issues-dismissed-for-misconduct

Glossary

Disability Evaluation System (DES): This refers generally to disability evaluation, including both the current Integrated Disability Evaluation System (IDES) and the Legacy Disability Evaluation System (LDES).

Integrated Disability Evaluation System (IDES): This refers to the system that has been in effect since 2012 when the DoD and VA disability evaluations were fully integrated. Between 2007 and 2011, pilots of an integrated system were conducted, so there is overlap between the Legacy Disability Evaluation System (LDES) and IDES.

Legacy Disability Evaluation System (LDES): This refers to system that was in effect prior to 2012, when the Integrated Disability Evaluation System (IDES) was fully implemented across DoD. LDES is still used currently on a case-by-case basis, as of 2015 when the Office of the Under Secretary of Defense (Personnel and Readiness) issued a memo about the use of the legacy system.

Medical/Disability Discharge: For the purposes of this report, medical/disability retirements and medical/disability separations are collectively referred to as *military/disability discharges*. In other words, a medical/disability discharge occurs when a service member is evaluated for disability and found unfit to continue serving, regardless of his or her disability rating.

Medical/Disability Retirement: Members who have been determined to be unfit for duty with a disability rated by the military Service as 30 percent or greater are eligible for disability retirement. (Source: https://militarypay.defense.gov/Pay/Retirement/Disability.aspx)

Medical/Disability Separation: Members who have been determined to be unfit for duty with a disability rated by the military service as less than 30 percent are eligible for disability separation.

Permanent Disability (Retired List): Members whose condition has stabilized at a disability rating of 30 percent or higher may be placed on the permanent disability retired list (PDRL). (U.S. Code, Title 10, Chapter 61)

Service-Connected Disability: This is an injury or illness that is incurred or aggravated during active military service. (Source: https://www.va.gov/opa/publications/benefits_book/benefits_chap02.asp)

Temporary Disability (Retired List): A member with a disability rating of 30 percent or higher whose condition is not stable may be placed on the temporary disability retired list (TDRL) for up to five years (three years as of 2017) at which point he or she must be either discharged, retired, or returned to duty. (U.S. Code, Title 10, Chapter 61)